The Serena Technique of Belly Dancing

The fun way to a trim shape

by
Serena and Alan Wilson

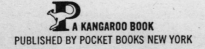

A KANGAROO BOOK
PUBLISHED BY POCKET BOOKS NEW YORK

THE SERENA TECHNIQUE OF BELLY DANCING

Drake edition published January, 1973

POCKET BOOK edition published January, 1974

This POCKET BOOK edition includes every word contained in
the original, higher-priced edition. It is printed from brand-
new plates made from completely reset, clear, easy-to-read type.
POCKET BOOK editions are published by
POCKET BOOKS,
a Simon & Schuster Division of
GULF & WESTERN CORPORATION
1230 Avenue of the Americas,
New York, N.Y. 10020.
Trademarks registered in the United States
and other countries.

4587

SLIM DOWN

THE FUN, CREATIVE WAY

If you've always wanted to get in shape, look more attractive, and feel healthier—without the dull routine of calisthenics—then this is the book for you.

In **THE SERENA TECHNIQUE OF BELLY DANCING,** Serena gives you the same lessons she's given to thousands of students who have passed through her enormously popular New York studio. You'll love practicing the graceful motions; they're guaranteed to make you feel 100 percent woman! And almost before you know it, you'll be noticeably slimmer and fitter.

Belly dancing is also great for posture and flexibility, a confidence-building creative outlet, and the oldest known way of preparing for natural childbirth. It is an art form with something to offer every woman—so why not start enjoying it today?

DEDICATION

Dedicated to the memory of my parents,
whose active participation in all the arts, created
the atmosphere and mood of my own private world.

Serena

CONTENTS

How to Use This Book 11

Introduction 13

The History of the Belly Dance 21

Specific Benefits of the Dance 40

    Getting the Most out of the Dance 40

    Exercise 44

    Advanced Routines 223

Getting Started 58

The Warm-up 61

Beginner Steps 84

    Beginner Routines 110

Intermediate Steps 112

    Intermediate Routines 153

Advanced Steps 155

    Advanced Routine 223

Appendix I: Music 229

Appendix II: Costumes 237

Appendix III: Putting on a Show 243

Appendix IV: Exercise Chart 247

Index of Steps 253

BODY CHART

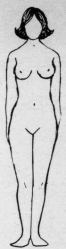

1-Normal

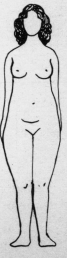

*4-Belly
and
Thigh
Thickness*

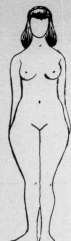

*2-Riding
Breeches
Type*

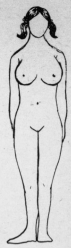

*3-Shoulder
and
Breast
Bigness*

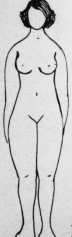

*5-Large
Extremities*

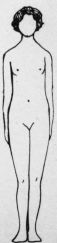

6-Juvenile

HOW TO USE
THIS BOOK

You will get maximum benefits from the dance if you follow the outline below:

1. Read and think about all the chapters up to the Warm-Up.

2. Learn the warm-up steps in order. Once you know them all, run through the entire warm-up routine, doing the steps as instructed. These steps are intended for everyone and are a good general exercise schedule all by themselves. Do the warm-up steps at the beginning of each practice session regardless of your specific needs. In doing them for the first time, you will quickly discover what special exercises you need.

3. Study the Body Type Chart on the facing page, and find the figure which best matches yours. Remember that the illustrations show the distribution of fat that is natural according to the hereditary characteristics of the woman pictured. The chart indicates the *tendency* of fat to accumulate in certain areas, and this tendency is inherited. Once you have found your general body type and have decided on which of the available benefits you need, turn to Appendix IV, where you will find an outline of the steps best suited to you. Do *not* skip around in the book! Learn all the steps you can, in the order they are given, but never overdo! Observe all caution notes, and do not attempt movements that are beyond you.

4. As you learn, place emphasis on the steps you need most, but don't ignore others in doing so. Don't forget to do the warm-up steps before each practice session, as you may be too "cold" to get full benefits from the ones you need.

5. If you intend to dance before an audience, refer to the costume section (Appendix II), and start planning ahead for a costume. You should have a practice skirt and veil by the time you get to the advanced section.

INTRODUCTION

Questions and Answers

One of the pleasures of the students at my studio is the daily gab session we have before and after classes. They enjoy letting their hair down, pouring a cup of coffee, and just talking about the dance, and themselves, and asking me questions. During these sessions, I am not a teacher on a platform in the classroom; I am a friend with whom they can discuss their problems on a give-and-take basis. Even though I hope to be a friend to you, the reader, I will be a teacher in this book and will not have the opportunity to discuss things with you or answer your questions directly. So I have decided that instead of writing a long-winded introduction in glowing praise of the dance, I will take this chance to give some straightforward answers to questions most asked by beginning students, just as I do in person.

QUESTION: If the belly dance is so ancient, why do you call your technique *new?*
ANSWER: Our language is old, too, but that doesn't mean we can't write anything new with it! To me, the dance is a language. It is a means of expression. I have chosen the dance as my way to self-expression because it represents the qualities of poise, grace, stamina, femininity, and an

13

enormous challenge to free creativity. When I say free creativity, I mean that the movements are *natural* to a woman rather than distorted and artificial as they are in ballet. The technique I have created is *mine,* just as Shakespeare's plays are *his*. Words were in existence long before Shakespeare used them, but what he created was *new*. Women danced the belly dance thousands of years before I came along, but what I have done with the steps is *new*. Actually, my dance shouldn't be called the belly dance at all, but it *is* a version of it, and since the term is so well known, I'll let it stand . . . at least for awhile.

QUESTION: Then, if this is your technique, how can you call it *authentic* belly dancing?

ANSWER: What I call it depends on who I am talking to, and what their definition of *authentic* is. Some people cling to the foolish logic that since much of the dance comes from Turkey, it must be true that the only authentic dancers are Turkish. Nothing could be further from the truth. All of the Turkish dancers I know learned the dance right here in the U.S.A. As a matter of fact, a very prominent dancer told me that she seldom heard Turkish music until she came to this country . . . she listened to American jazz on her radio in Turkey!

There is a difference between *authentic* and *genuine*. Authentic means *true,* or the *opposite of false*. To me the dance is creativity, the growth of ideas and imagination. I consider myself authentic because I am true to its spirit and principles rather than what it has always been in terms of steps and routines. On the other hand, my dance is not *genuine* in the sense that it is a carbon-copy of someone else's movements . . . whether these movements were done yesterday, or a thousand years ago. I don't consider the dance to be an Olympic Game to see who can jump the highest, split the widest, or do what she is told most exactly.

Many of my steps are traditional, and they are so beautiful that I wouldn't dream of changing them. But the blend and interpretation are mine, and I never perform without Middle Eastern music. I might add that I perform almost exclusively for Middle Eastern audiences, and my authenticity has never been challenged.

QUESTION: Since the dance is really a performing art, why do you say it is a physical fitness program?
ANSWER: I don't. I still say it is a performing art, the same as I say baseball is a sport, not a profession. Many more people play baseball for the fun of it than for money; and many more women dance for the pleasure and other benefits than enter show business as a career. According to my records, 87 per cent of my students are studying the dance because they enjoy it, *and* for the excellent exercise value. They range in age from 7 to 75, and come from every walk of life: housewives, secretaries, lawyers, college students, clerks, even an oceanographer who is probably the first and only woman to belly dance at the South Pole! Of the remaining 13 per cent, less than one per cent ever go on to dance professionally. Of course, performing doesn't mean making a career of it. Many women get great pleasure out of dancing at social functions of organizations they belong to, and at parties in their homes. For this reason, there are sections on party-giving (with menu and decorating ideas) and a costume section for those of you who would like to make one. Of course, there are also plenty of hints for the professional, as well as outlines for fully professional routines . . . nothing is left out!

Belly dancing has always been a *functional* dance. By this I mean that it has always had a practical *reason to be*. It was used in fertility rites, and was the first exercise regimen for natural childbirth. It has been used to make women more attractive sexually, and has been awarded a role in sex education. As the centuries have passed, it has been adapted to the needs at hand. New steps and movements were added as they were required. I have collected these steps, added some of my own, and this book is the result . . . the only book ever published which contains them. There are 88 different steps, 119 variations, 146 combinations, and 67 challenge combinations (for the ambitious)! That's 420 different movements!

I don't know of a better system of exercise, but I didn't deliberately make it that way. The benefits are built into the steps themselves; the art came first, and the exercise value followed as part of it.

In keeping with my belief that the dance should serve the best interests of today's woman, I have carefully catalogued the steps and analyzed their value, so that you can determine what benefits you need, and then go about getting them with a minimum of effort and confusion.

Now, it's up to *you* to decide. Is it art or exercise? Or both? Perhaps you would prefer a new name for it. Exerdance? Articise? Call it what you will, it's a lot of fun, and you'll get a lot out of it!

QUESTION: You mentioned sex; isn't the belly dance really a sex dance?

ANSWER: I remember being taught, in an English class in college, that there are only two basic subjects in art: sex and religion. The belly dance embraces both, and the effect depends on your interpretation and the emphasis you place on it. But if the dance is only *sexy,* then it stops being belly dancing and becomes stripping or exotic dancing, and certainly bears no relation to my technique.

Very often, it isn't what something *is,* it's what you *call* it that counts. For example, there is a very delicious fish that comes from the Gulf of Mexico, and it is commonly known as "red snapper." Tasty as it is, it just simply wouldn't sell under that name, so a clever promoter changed the name to "ocean perch." The fish immediately became a gourmet delight, and is now a commercial success. And how about the girl with the awful voice who could never sell her singing, but is a sensation as a "song stylist"? Even janitors aren't janitors any more . . . they're *sanitation engineers!* Acceptance goes with the proper title.

Unfortunately, the term "belly dance" reminds us of carnivals, and Coney Island, the antics of Little Egypt (of the 1890's), and the foolish interpretation of Hollywood movies. Even though I don't compare myself to the fish, or the stylist, or the janitor, as a professional performer and as a teacher, I can't overlook the prejudices of the consumer. Belly dancing has the reputation of being sexy, and there is nothing I can do about it—except to change the name, which is exactly what I do. When I know that the term *belly dancer* might cause eyebrows to raise, I become an *oriental dancer.* Same costume, same music, same performance . . . but now it is alright for the most sedate audience to rest easy because I'm not a belly dancer any more!

The belly dance isn't sexy—it is *sensual,* and there is a big difference between the two. A sexy dance is random flesh-peddling. Any woman can do it. It takes no special skill or artistry; all she needs is her natural equipment. It is the same as the difference between pornography and erotic literature: pornography serves only to arouse; eroticism has the depth of romance. But this is a subject that is discussed later in the book, and I don't want to dwell on it here. However, I can say that your approach to the dance, as modified by your philosophical beliefs as well as your skill, will determine to what extent sex plays a part in your performance.

I have danced for audiences where even the slightest trace of lewdness or vulgarity would have been out of place: a missionary group at Riverside Church in New

York; Mayor Lindsay in the New York City Council Chambers as part of an International Cultural Program; the Women's American ORT. The steps in this book are just as I performed them for these groups, and just as I teach them in class. I do my full show in all its sensuous aspects, and am accepted as an artist, not *in spite of* my sensuality, but *because* of it.

QUESTION: I have seen belly dancers that I thought were vulgar. How do you define vulgarity?

ANSWER: If I were to embark on a great philosophical discussion of vulgarity in the light of all the constantly changing moral standards, we would never get on with this book, and you would never start dancing! So for the sake of brevity and accuracy, I have my own definition of vulgarity by which I measure the dance:

> *vulgarity:* reduction of the sensual to the sexual; distortion of dance steps resulting in a coarse and common expression of sex.

It is the *suggestion* of sex—the *implication,* not the indiscriminate promise, of new and mysterious wonders—which give the dance the fascination it holds. Outright sexual movements are not mysterious; in fact, they are so commonly known that they are nothing more than a biological display. But they are easy to perform because, after all, they are natural to all of us. For this reason, it is common for bad dancers (or dancers who refuse to spend the time and energy to learn to dance well) to go into the obscenity business. The result doesn't deserve comment.

QUESTION: Now that I know something about it, what can the dance do for me?

ANSWER: That is the subject of this book . . . read on, enjoy yourself, and good luck!

SERENA
September, 1972

The Serena Technique of Belly Dancing

THE HISTORY
OF THE BELLY DANCE

Is it possible that the first dance ever done by a woman was the belly dance? If we could peer back through the haze of time and secretly watch our cave sister, what kind of a dance do you think she would be doing? The belly dance, of course!

Here's why we think so: The dance is an art; it is a means of expression, which is another way of saying it is a means of communication. Whenever we communicate with one another (or with God, as in religious dances), we express the thoughts and ideas that interest us most at the time. Now, it's reasonable to believe that the first women had two basic interests: food and sex. We know this because there are many ancient artifacts which tell us so. For example, there are rock engravings of ritual fertility dances in the Cave of Addaura, near Palermo in Sicily, which date back 15,000 years before Christ. Hunting also is a dominant theme, though this activity seems more confined to men, with the women satisfied to do the eating.

As centuries passed, the dance developed and gained in popularity with artists, appearing in Egyptian tomb paintings as early as 5000 B.C. and in ancient Greek sculpture. Probably, the greatest interest in the dance as a subject for sculpture was displayed in our own century during the Art Nouveau period as is evidenced by the magnificent bronzes in Serena's collection.

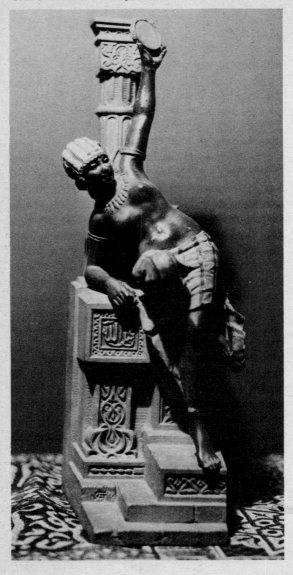

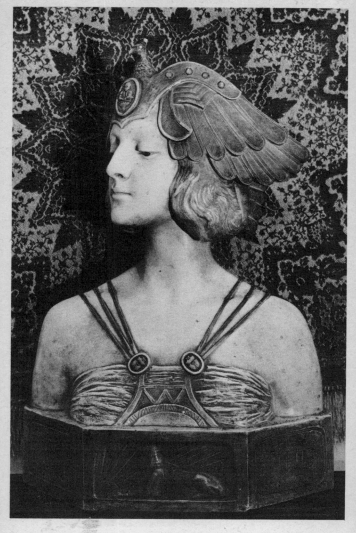

Statues in Serena's Collection

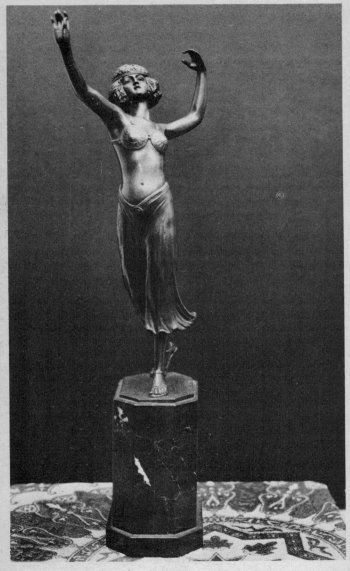

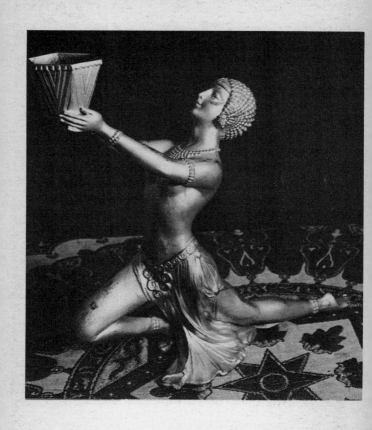

Statues in Serena's Collection

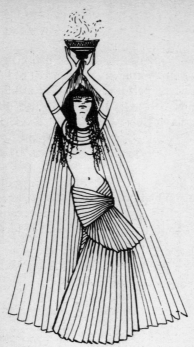

We know that the early dances were so devoted to sex that they would undoubtedly be considered obscene by today's standards. Yet morality shifts with the demands of the time, and it would be foolish as well as pointless to make moral judgments of an art which endures well beyond the flexibility of our rules of right and wrong.

The concept of fertility, and of course the sexual activity necessary to make it practical, is a basic concern in any religion. The attitude of a people is indicated in its attempts to control natural functions, *i.e.,* the prohibitions placed upon them by their religion.

In an attempt to discover just what a natural function is and to see how such a function manifested itself as physical expression we performed an experiment. Using a wide variety of people, we took them aside, one at a time, and asked them to assume postures which they thought would best describe such things as hate, suspicion, greed, anger, love. Then we took the postures produced by our experimental subjects, performed them for a different group, and asked them to identify them. It turned out that there *were* absolute similarities, and that good understanding of abstractions could be achieved by movements alone. The differences among people were expressed by their degree of inhibition.

There is no doubt that much of what they did depended on conditioning. Which means they *learned* their responses from watching them on TV, stage, and movies. Anger triggered a scowl, while satisfaction produced a smile.

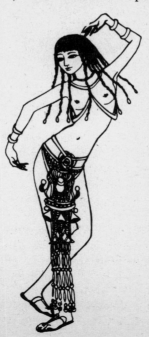

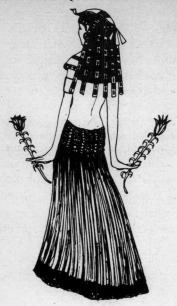

Each reaction was directly related to movements naturally involved in the act. Love and sex blended into motions of hugging, kissing, caressing . . . and obvious sexual actions.

Now, you might ask, "What does all this have to do with belly dancing?" The answer is that in exploring the history of the dance we are not so much interested in minute details, as we are in *why* they did it, and how belly dancing evolved as a purely natural art rather than a contrived one.

The blacks of Central Africa used the belly dance as a means of sexual selection; the girls danced for the men, directing their attentions to their favorites . . . and the men made their choices. In Loango the dance is devoted to the worship of ancestors and future generations, the idea being the transmission of life. The Cambodians employed snakelike movements; in the Celebe, the abdominal dance was called *masseri,* meaning Egyptian. The daughters of Jerusalem performed a kind of fertility dance in the vineyards which was ecstatic and frenzied.

The belly dance was described variously as "abdominal dances," "hip dances with considerable rolling of pelvises," and even as "posterior dances." Though it is beyond us to do so here, it would make an interesting study as to *why* the dance appeared *where* it did. Did the dance develop on its own in these countries, or was it carried by wandering tribes and explorers? If it arose spontaneously, why did it appear where it did? Why, for instance, isn't it performed in India, which has a rich tradition of erotica? It would certainly make a fascinating study through which we would learn a great deal about ourselves.

The way the belly dance originated has never been discovered fully, to anyone's satisfaction. There is still dis-

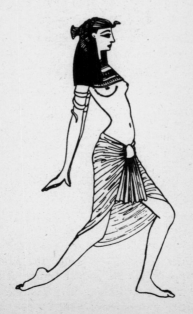

agreement as to how the dance got to Egypt. Officials at the Egyptian Ministry of Culture and National Guidance attribute the dance to the Turks, who ruled Egypt for 400 years. Another Egyptian authority admits that the finger-bells were introduced into Egypt by the Turks, but claims that the dance was originated by the Phoenicians. We believe that the dance probably originated in Persia, at the same time as the development of the *oud* (predecessor of the lute), and moved toward the Mediterranean, splitting off to go into Egypt on the south, and to Turkey to the north.

An interesting relic of the dance is the practice of the *awalem*. These are dancers who, standing in one place, perform highly sexual movements for the purpose of instructing the uninitiated in sexual matters. Most weddings employed two or three of them, and even today wealthy couples will have a dancer at their matrimonial celebrations in order to preserve the tradition.

The belly dance was almost unknown in the United States until 1893, when Little Egypt and her dancers appeared at the Chicago World's Fair and gave Victorian audiences a shock from which they never recovered. Belly dancing was here to stay!

Little Egypt was neither little, nor Egyptian. Her real name was Fahreda Mahzar, and she was Syrian. But statistics didn't concern the happy fair-goers. A trip to the World's Fair was synonymous with seeing Little Egypt . . . and see her they did. "Every muscle in her body at the same time," as they said. Eugene Field sang her praises, first in describing "Moorish maidens with bangles of gold" and concluding with, "And hush, we'll see that Algerian dance—Come boys, let's away to the Midway Plaisance."

According to all accounts, Little Egypt and her friends were not very good dancers. A souvenir book of the fair had this to say: "Of the performance it may be said that

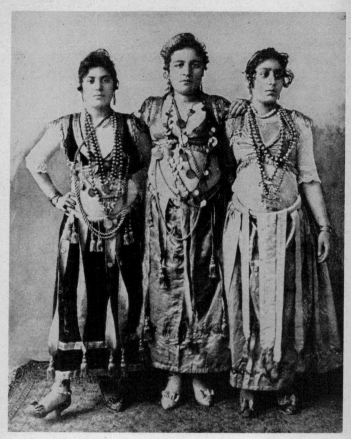

Egyptian Dancing Girls at the Worlds Fair of 1893

it was something entirely new in America and something not likely to become acclimatized. Suggestive it certainly was, but to American eyes lacked even the redeeming quality of beauty, though the dancers were lithe as panthers and should have been capable of graceful movements. . . . Their dancing is a profession to which they are trained from childhood though it can hardly be considered a dance so much as a contortion."

But the book goes on grudgingly to admit that the dancers were an instant success, and that their "contortions" attracted enormous crowds to the Midway Plaisance. Naturally, so popular an attraction could hardly escape the attention of the Board of Lady Managers, who immediately pressured the director general to demand that future exhibitions be restrained "within the limits of stage propriety as recognized in this country."

Fortunately, motion pictures were taken of Little Egypt's dance. Not so fortunate is the fact her mid-section was nearly obliterated by the black stripes of the censor. What does remain shows only a few harmless gyrations by a heavily draped woman.

If the dance were only "vulgarly appealing" as the book says, it was also a box-office bonanza. Whatever "restraints" were applied at the fair, they were certainly ignored by the owners of vaudeville houses. Plaisance Dancers, named after the Midway Plaisance, appeared on burlesque stages across the country, and were a smashing success. Catherine Devine, who claimed to be the original Little Egypt, rode the crest of the craze until her death in 1908, when her Coney Island imitators moved in to capitalize on her popularity.

Little Egypt herself may have been a fraud, and there is good reason to think she was, but the Dancing Girls were certainly Syrian. The dance they did was probably a collection of traditional folk steps which reflected a life and culture very different from ours. It's also possible that

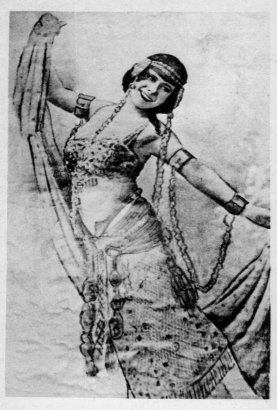

Little Egypt

their movements were not graceful, at least by American standards of 1893 in which women and corsets and rigidity were synonymous. It didn't occur to the reporter at the fair that if the situation were reversed, the Egyptian visitors might have found our painted society ladies "suggestive" and "vulgar"!

But there was an odd moral atmosphere at the time. Victorian standards were beginning to disintegrate. Realizing that it would be impossible to enforce them on a grand scale, the crusaders of the faith stopped trying to influence the lower classes, whom they considered to be a lost cause anyway, and doubled their efforts to purify the cultural air breathed by those who counted in society. The riff-raff were left to wallow in the degradations of Chicago's tenderloin, while the police, goaded by reformers, censured the content of legitimate stage productions for profane or offensive language. Apparently the sensitivities of the Chicago police were highly developed, for numerous performances were stopped until scripts were rewritten.

This spirit of righteousness prevailed in the Chicago of 1910, when on November 25 the great Mary Garden appeared in the opera *Salome*. Her Dance of the Seven Veils stunned the audience and exploded into a rage of controversy. Fearful that the sterling morals of the Windy City were in jeopardy, the chief of police hurried to the second performance, which had already been sold out.

Leroy T. Steward, Chicago's chief of police and erudite protector of the public morals, thought the show was disgusting. He couldn't see any art in her dance, and if there were any art at all, it must have been "Black Art." He compared Miss Garden's dance to a cat wallowing in a bed of catnip. It might have been interesting to compare Mr. Steward's review of the opera with that of the New York police, but in keeping with New York's progressive thinking, the show had already been banned there.

To avoid the unpleasantness of an officially enforced

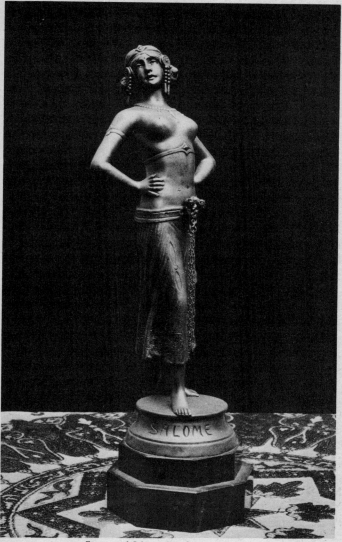

Statue of Mary Garden as Salome

closing, the management of the opera ended its run voluntarily. Miss Garden was furious. She protested that her dance was inspired and beautiful, and besides, she never bared her tummy, and she didn't roll it as was done in the hoochi-kooch she had seen in Algiers.

Salome didn't die in Chicago. Miss Garden went on, with her dance, and her flowing pink veils, to Milwaukee where she performed and was accepted without complaint. Whether the people in Milwaukee were more sophisticated than Chicagoans or whether they just pretended to be doesn't really matter; what does matter is that they had watched Mary Garden wallow in her bed of catnip and showed no visible signs of moral corruption.

Of course, strippers and exotics were quick to adopt the idea of the Seven Veils. Many of them became belly dancers overnight, enjoying the touch of art they injected into their performances, along with the extra benefit that a few dollars' worth of veils constituted an easily removable wardrobe.

This invasion of the art by opportunistic flesh peddlers produced the tawdry sexual image that stigmatizes the dance even today. Serious dancers, who saw great possibilities in Oriental dancing, resented the term belly dance preferring instead *danse du ventre* with the hope that anything French might add a veneer of class. Actually, neither of the terms is correct, nor is *abdominal dance* as used by some historians, since the belly plays a very small part in the dance as we know it. Most artists avoid calling it anything at all, and simply use the steps without giving credit where it's due.

The popularity of the dance focused attention on the Middle East, whose rich culture, dormant for centuries, offered a wealth of unexploited possibilities. A colorful variety of mysterious and exotic products appeared on the market. Advertising claims based on secret Oriental ingredients, or hinting at sexual pleasure, impressed an

American public steeped to the limit in Puritan stuffiness. The merchandise ranged from an Egyptian pile cure to perfumes, and even an Arabian joint oil, but the cigarette manufacturers outdid all the others in vividly portraying the exotic naughtiness of the Middle East. In 1896, a year in which women were discouraged from smoking at all and certainly never puffed in public, there appeared an ad for Ateshian Turkish Cigarets. An Oriental dancing girl, wearing a low-cut halter bedangled with jewels and coins, sheer pantaloons, veils, and bare tummy sat cross-legged on a Persian rug casually holding an Ateshian Cigaret and ecstatically blowing a stream of smoke from her lips! The implications were obvious, and stirred many women to dangerous thoughts and secret daydreams.

It was just such an advertising poster for Egyptian Deities Cigarettes, complete with the goddess Isis sitting on her throne beside the river Nile, that inspired the child who was to become one of the greatest interpretive dancers this country has ever known: Ruth St. Denis.

She danced her first professional performance as an Oriental dancer at Proctor's Twenty-third Street Theater in New York in 1906. We can only imagine how the idealistic young girl, who considered herself to be the embodiment of Egyptian mystery and beauty, felt as her dance was sandwiched in between Bob Fitzsimmons, the boxer, and a herd of trained monkeys.

Undaunted, but leery of prize-fighters and performing apes, Miss St. Denis rented a theater specifically for her dance, and performed before a select group. The next day her performance was reviewed in the *New York Telegraph* as a "Wow! A mixture of hoochee-koochee and Cake Walk. What matter if the movements of the torso below the short jacket divulged every undulation of the flesh? It was all quite as much as the most daring had anticipated." Still another critic thought her dance interpreted beautiful things and could be as expressive as music and poetry. All of which makes us wonder about the wisdom of listening to critics at all!

Miss St. Denis could have at least elevated her critical acclaim out of the hoochee-koochee and cake walk category if she had chosen ballet. But she, as well as her more volatile contemporary Isadora Duncan, had little regard for ballet. Neither liked the sterile and confining orthodoxy of it, but Miss Duncan was the more outspoken: "Those who enjoy it see no farther than the skirts and tricots, but look under the skirts, under the tricots are dancing deformed muscles. Look still further; underneath the muscles are deformed bones. A deformed skeleton is dancing before you. This deformation through incorrect dress and incorrect movement is the result of the learning necessary to the ballet. The ballet condemns itself by enforcing the deformation of the beautiful woman's body. No historical, no choreographic reasons can prevail against that!"

Strong words from Miss Duncan! But were they true or just sour grapes? Both dancers preached the naturalness, the healthful benefits, the creative expression, the femininity, the sensuality, and the freedom of Oriental dancing. Miss Duncan said, "The dancer of the future will dance the freedom of woman . . . the highest intelligence in the freest body."

While the *Boston Sunday Herald* proclaimed that Ruth St. Denis "could dance wholly undraped and be the incarnation of unconscious purity," the Middle East, cradle of the dance, was converting the old dance to the cabaret version we know today.

In 1927 the Casino Opera in Cairo became *the* birthplace of modern belly dancing in Egypt. At first the dancers performed in a chorus line, but those with real talent soon went out on their own.

Meanwhile, back in Greece, the Turkish street dancers were still dancing for coins tossed at them by admiring spectators. With visions of golden streets in their heads, many came to this country to perform, bringing with them the custom of tipping, just in case. Today if you visit a real Greek nightclub, you will see bills of all denominations (never coins!) plastered to the dancer's moist body, or showered upon her by an appreciative audience.

As an illustration of how widely practiced belly dancing is today, many women's organizations invite Serena to lecture on and demonstrate the dance at their meetings. In order to give them first-hand experience in the dance, she gives them a short beginner's lesson. They enjoy participating as a group, partly because their enthusiasm is contagious, and partly because learning a new art is more fun if you share the experience with others. As a result, they form dance exercise groups just as they do for card games or sports. They hold their practice sessions at each other's homes and have the fun and excitement of doing the steps together in a party atmosphere.

Occasionally, after they have become proficient enough in the dance, they sponsor a dinner-dance or banquet on a Middle Eastern theme at which they perform. Such social functions make excellent fund-raising affairs for religious or civic groups. If you enjoy participating in group activities, such an organization might be for you!

Now we have another page in the history of the dance with the Serena Technique; blending the old with the new; searching for the natural and ultimate truth of woman. But this is where we came in . . . now it's your turn to write some history!

SPECIFIC BENEFITS
OF THE DANCE

Getting the Most out of the Dance

This book presents the dance as an art form, and if you seriously set out to master all the steps, you *could* become an expert performer. However, Oriental dancing, more than other dance forms, has developed qualities which benefit the performer as well as entertain an audience.

People love to dance, and according to cave paintings that are thousands of years old, they always have. In fact, since movement is the most basic form of self-expression, it's more than likely that people danced before they had music to accompany them. From religious observances to war dances, from fertility rites to festivals, it's hard to imagine a civilization without its dances.

Dancing has survived as an art because people enjoy doing it. It's not only a means of communicating a story, an idea, or a mood; it's also physically satisfying as well. It can build you to a pitch of excitement, or it can release your tensions and relax you into calmness and serenity. It can make you think, or it can transport you beyond thought. It can heighten your senses and awareness of yourself, or it can vaporize all material things and leave you alone with the spiritual. It is nature and life and, most important, it is whatever you want it to be. As you learn the steps in this book, you will be learning a vocabulary of movements, a language from which you will write your own poetry; and your creations will be uniquely yours.

Part of the Serena Technique is based on traditional folk steps which have evolved through centuries of Middle Eastern culture. Most of them are easy to do, and you will find that in a very short time, you will know enough steps to enjoy putting a basic dance together.

These folk steps are intended to be done by all women regardless of age or body type. (It is assumed that women with medical problems will consult their physicians before engaging in *any* kind of physical exertion.) One of the joys of the movements is that though each is designed as an exercise to benefit the dancer, the audience is never aware of it! Whether you have selected a sequence of steps to trim your waistline, increase your sense of balance, or improve your posture, you will still be performing a very exciting and graceful dance.

The specific exercise value of the various steps is discussed elsewhere in this book, but it cannot be stressed enough that in order for you to get *full exercise value,* you must do the steps exactly as they are described and illustrated. There are enough steps in each group so that if you find one that does not appeal to you aesthetically or is not for your body type, simply select another with the same benefits. It is *never* necessary or desirable to plod through steps which don't interest you or which you don't like. Remember that your practice sessions should be *fun;* don't turn them into dull routines of calisthenics which would tempt you to cheat. It is the monotony of most exercise systems that causes people to abandon them. Furthermore, many women find that most of the common exercises are unattractive and masculine.

You will learn a great deal about yourself as you go along. You will become increasingly aware of your body: what it looks like, how it works, and what its capabilities are. You will probably discover a you that you didn't know existed. Don't be afraid to criticize yourself, but be honest in both directions—good as well as bad. Genuine confidence is impossible without a realistic appraisal of yourself. If you believe that you have done a step especially well, tell yourself so, out loud! Applaud yourself when you deserve it. At the same time, throw away your rose-colored glasses. If you see a stiff, awkward woman in your mirror, admit it and do something about it. After all, you owe it to the dance as well as to yourself to give it your best, and that means the most graceful and attractive *you* that you can create.

You will probably find that you are better than you thought you would be. You will want more of a challenge than the simple folk steps have to offer. To meet this need, there are many steps which are difficult; some are *very* strenuous, and others require such exceptional skill that they would challenge any professional dancer in any dance form. However, don't feel compelled to try these steps just because they are there. By the time you feel ready for greater challenge, you will have a reasonably good idea of your individual abilities. At this point, it's wise to consider the economist's advice: Live a little beyond your means; it makes you work harder. In other words, bite off a *little* more than you can chew; perfect each step you select, *don't skip,* but always have your eye on the next step.

Once you have selected your steps, forget that you are exercising. The benefits will be there whether you know it or not. Concentrate on the emotional content of the steps you are doing, and try to create the frame of mind which suits you best at the moment. There is a wide variety of moods to choose from: the pensive, sensuous cifte telli; the almost outrageous joy of the Turkish Kashlimar; the solemn fluidity of a taksim, or the unrestrained seductiveness of the undulations. Whatever you choose, express yourself completely. Let yourself go, and release your emotions through your movements. You will be surprised at the results!

This dance is closely associated with sex, and rightly so. Though never vulgar, as it is when performed by its exploiters, the movements are highly sensuous and can be sexually stimulating. This is one of the natural characteristics of the dance which have remained through the centuries and which have a natural wholesomeness.

The dance was once performed in pagan fertility rites and was considered useful in preparing for natural childbirth. It seemed to be effective in both respects, though there is some question as to whether the gods were responsible for the fertility, or whether men found the women more attractive when they danced!

The steps are not intended to directly enhance sexual performance, though there is no doubt that both increased body tone and abdominal and pelvic strength and flexibility would contribute to it.

The dance is sexually stimulating. It may surprise you though to know that the dance is stimulating both to the man who watches it and to the woman who performs it! A woman who is capable of arousing herself is also attractive and arousing to men as an entire being rather than just as a sexual toy.

In all respects, one of the great values of the dance is the discovery and development of the whole self—which includes increased self-confidence and femininity. Many pretty women are often surprised and dismayed to often find themselves passed by in favor of their much plainer sisters. True sexual beauty and desirability are generated by the natural qualities of complete femininity rather than by artificial appearance or mechanical technique which lacks sincerity.

Age is a problem faced by all women. The older woman wants youth without the awkwardness and inexperience that go with it. How many times have you heard people say, "Oh, if I could only be twenty years younger, and still know what I know today!"? The teen-ager wants poise and maturity without the wrinkles. Dancing provides the control and grace necessary to eliminate awkwardness as well as the exercise needed to tone the body, but just as important, it inspires the interested enthusiasm which is the essence of ageless youth. There is no need to abandon all of the charms and pleasures of childhood because of the number of years you have lived. An active, interested, enthusiastic, flexible woman is *young*. A girl of sixteen is *old* if she loses interest in herself and in life; a woman of seventy-five is *young* if she retains it.

So pamper yourself a little. Be a little selfish. As you learn the steps and practice them, spend some time getting to know yourself. Take advantage of all you have to offer. Instead of just thinking beautiful, *be beautiful naturally*. People will love you for it.

Exercise

Professional promoters of exercise systems and owners of "Spas" and posh Health Clubs are well aware of the reluctance of the average, busy woman to exercise, so they are quick to sugar-coat their methods with elegant surroundings, tropical lagoons, and glistening machines as though exercise were on a par with a painful trip to the dentist. But have you ever noticed that they never tell you what exercise really is?

The word *exercise* simply means to *use*. For example, if you *exercise* your right to vote, it means that you are *using* it. If you *exercise* your body, which you do every time you move it, you are *using* it. Obviously, just because you are using it doesn't mean that you are doing it any particular good, any more than practicing using a voting machine will guarantee that you will cast a ballot for the best candidate. It is necessary to use physical exercise intelligently.

Unfortunately, exercise has the reputation of being work. A session at the gym is often called a workout. Judging from the number of people enrolled at gymnasiums, there are many who enjoy work, and there is no doubt that the kind of physical exertion done in gymnastics and athletics can be beneficial. However, there are also many people who don't like that kind of work yet who torture themselves with exercises they don't really need . . . *because of the very unpleasantness of it!* They seem to feel that anything which is painful must per se be good for them, just as the nastiest tasting medicine is always thought to be the most effective.

Gymnastics and calisthenics have their benefits: the development of skill; physical strength and stamina; a curiosity about and a respect for the body and its functions. Belly dancing, while being much more enjoyable, also incorporates these same benefits. Amid all the other fads—food fads, odd diets, "exercise" machines, health religions—it's good for a chuckle to note that belly dancing has also been called a fad. If it's true, then the women who have been enjoying it for the past several thousand years have been participating in the world's longest-running temporarily popular art!

The dance also provides us with the kind of make-believe or role-playing you enjoy in wearing a new dress or changing your make-up and hair style. It gives you a chance to act out the many facets of your personality.

You might ask, What does role-playing have to do with exercise? If we were discussing bar-bells and rowing machines, the answer would be, Nothing! But the dance is an art. It requires creative imagination; it involves *thought*. You will not be one of many robots doing the same movement the same way, over and over again. The dance *is* life, with all the variety of energy and emotion life has to offer. You will find that your experiences, both physical and emotional, in the dance will become a powerful influence in your life.

Our bodies are seldom called upon to perform all the functions of which they are capable. Unfortunately, the demand for full capability often comes in the form of an emergency, and we are not always up to meeting it. This is one of the reasons Serena has developed her technique of the dance. We would have little need for exercise if we were able to engage in all the activities we were designed for. But, in order to do so, it would be necessary to regress to the most primitive existence. Few of us would be willing to give up our modern conveniences, especially when we remember that of the first twenty-four pioneer women to arrive in this country only nine survived the first winter.

We haven't the time, resources, or the inclination to chase animals for food, swim rivers to catch fish, climb trees to gather fruit, and so on. Yet we were *designed* to do these things, and we have survived because we were (and are) able to do them. We have chosen to live a more comfortable and secure life, and whatever we take we must pay for . . . in this case with the condition of our bodies.

The dance as Serena presents it tones the entire body by exercising *all* of it. In addition to the more visible benefits, such as weight loss and flexibility, the dance has the effect (as have most athletic sports) of sharpening the senses, or faculties. For example, the sense of balance and control is greatly increased. At first this may seem to be a minor advantage to you, especially since you have no immediate plans to walk a tight-rope over Grand Canyon, but you do want to move gracefully and be sure-footed. This makes a great deal of sense when you consider that the vast majority of accidents occur in and around the home. We can only speculate as to how many falls could have been avoided if the victim had had a better sense of balance.

We find among the reasons to take up belly dancing some expected benefits and some surprising ones. You have probably already thought of the exercise and artistry, and probably even your increased awareness of yourself as a woman, but who would have suspected safety as a benefit?

Additional Benefits

Up to this point we have discussed the general benefits of the dance. The development of poise, balance, stamina, and physical strength are qualities we all want to have. Such qualities are the result of a well-planned and diversified program. However, it is possible to select steps, or routines, or even a mental attitude toward the dance, so that emphasis is placed on a specific area with a specific goal in mind. When definite parts of the dance are used to produce a prescribed effect, it then becomes therapy.

Recently, many physicians and psychiatrists have become aware of belly dancing as therapy, and have prescribed it as part of their treatment for a variety of disorders. The following outline is a very general discussion of some of the instances in which they have used it successfully. It is *not* a recommendation that you embark upon a regimen of self-treatment. However, if you should feel that you have a problem similar to one discussed below, by all means take this book to your physician for his advice.

PHYSICAL

To a great extent, our well-being and appearance depend on muscle tone and the absence of excess fat. It's well established that proper exercise and diet will aid the normal woman in achieving a trim, healthy body. Most women who dance for exercise do so for these cosmetic and hygienic reasons. Yet, strangely enough, fat is considered beautiful in many parts of the Middle East where the dance originated, and you will notice that most belly dancers are pictured as roly-poly if not downright fat. (In the travel section of the *New York Times,* Feb. 20, 1972, dancers in Istanbul were described as "forty pounds overweight.") The reasons for this are twofold: *(1)* The dance as they perform it does not specifically cause weight loss —which is another reason to prefer the Serena approach as opposed to strict authenticity! *(2)* In the Middle East, there is social status as well as aesthetic value in being plump, so rich foods are on the dancer's menu.

When you consider losing weight, or changing the contours of your body, you should be aware of the fact that the body you want may not be the body you should have. Your body type, and the distribution of fat, depend on many factors, not the least of which is heredity. Starvation diets, overwork or excessive exercise, or drugs to dull appetite or alter hormonal balance in order to produce a dream body that you were never intended to have in the first place can be extremely dangerous. When your doctor prescribes exercise of any kind, he intends for you to use it exactly as he directs, usually in combination with other treatment. If you go on the assumption of some students that, "If a little is good, then a lot must be better," and sneak in extra practice sessions, you can disrupt the entire program.

If you are practicing the dance conscientiously as directed, you will probably notice that you have trimmed down without the weight loss you might expect. You will also be aware of increased flexibility and mobility, and that you move with less effort, particularly when you bend, stoop, or reach. Because of this limbering effect, and because the exercise of the dance need only be as strenuous as you want it to be, physicians have recommended patients to Serena's studio for exercise. The following cases are representative of such referrals: *(1)* Patient A had suffered severe burns of the face, neck, and shoulder, and had undergone extensive skin-grafting; her doctor hoped that the movements of the dance would keep the skin flexible. *(2)* Patient B had undergone prosthesis of the hip joint (replacement of the natural joint with a plastic one) and attended classes (at first, on crutches) at the request of her orthopedist, who believed the dance might increase her ability to walk. *(3)* Several women were afflicted with back ailments such as herniated ("slipped") spinal discs. One orthopedist who had referred a patient is now seriously studying the possibility of using belly dance movements on male patients as well as female. He says that part of his interest in dance exercise is due to the fact that it is interesting and fun, and that patients are more apt to stay with it.

The list is extensive, and includes such diverse problems as the atrophy of muscles from polio, and coordination difficulties resulting from brain injury. But regardless of the success of belly dancing as therapy, it should be remembered that the cases described above were carefully selected by highly qualified medical men. Dancing will not cure a herniated disc, or cause paralyzed muscles to move, but the movements of the dance can be beneficial for certain physical problems and should not be overlooked as a therapeutic possibility.

EMOTIONAL

There is no doubt that emotional problems are responsible for the overwhelming majority of unhappy lives, especially when we realize that the way a person reacts toward his everyday difficulties can often be more damaging than the difficulty itself.

It may seem trite to say that a woman's attitude toward herself determines how happy she is, but sometimes the most obvious is the most apt to be overlooked, particularly in an age when we are looking for hidden meanings in everything. Even though we know the importance of attitude, we still don't know what a healthy attitude really is.

Psychiatrists estimate that we are "wrong," or technically incorrect, in two-thirds of what we say. It's no wonder that we create inaccurate and unrealistic evaluations of ourselves, and of the problems with which we are faced! We have trouble in deciding the magnitude of a problem and in measuring our ability to solve it. If we are presented with a difficult situation, and magnify that difficulty, while at the same time underestimating our ability to cope with it, then we find ourselves depressed and blue; the world seems bleak and grim. On the other hand, if we refuse to acknowledge the seriousness of a situation, and inflate ourselves with a false sense of competence, we are riding high on the road to disaster. In contrast to these extremes, the dance *forces* you to see yourself and your problems as they really are. Even though the problem may be no more than learning a dance step, you will have the opportunity to see yourself at work on intellectual and physical tasks that are actually smaller counterparts of the greater problems of life.

Today it is much too easy to avoid responsibility. If our jobs become too much for us, we can hide our mistakes in the anonymity of big business. If our TV set breaks down, we send for a serviceman. The act of making decisions and accepting the responsibility for them is one of the building blocks of maturity, and if the decision-making faculty is not used it deteriorates. The fact that so many women have allowed decisions to be made for them for so many years has resulted in their dependence on men. Awareness of this dependence is responsible for the rise of Women's Lib. Whether or not you agree with the principles of these groups, it must be admitted that they have brought attention to the problem. In this respect, there is probably no better way of exploring the meaning of femininity than through the dance.

The first step in sensible decision-making is a realistic appraisal of yourself, and the dance can be very effective in doing so. The second step is to understand the problem, and the dance can help here too. To see how the dance has helped others, let's consider the situations of some of Serena's students who came to her studio some time ago:

Student 1: Miss X had just been through a very unpleasant divorce. It left her bitter and disillusioned. She felt that she was no longer a desirable woman. She concealed her feeling of rejection by developing an overbearing and aggressive personality. She was a good secretary, but she lost job after job because of her bickering and domineering attitude. She came to the studio on the recommendation of a friend because she wanted the exercise. Once in the class, she couldn't escape her reflection in the mirror; she had to see herself as she really was. If she wanted to improve her image, she had to work at it. She discovered that the others in the class were so involved with themselves that no one noticed her or was critical of her, and that she had no one to impress or dominate. She began to take pride in her feminine self she saw emerging. She liked the genuine confidence she gained through learning to perform well. Men who had been avoiding her because of her righteous and competitive attitude began to notice her as a relaxed and very feminine woman. The phone, silent for so long, began to ring. She found that she could make decisions on a reasonable and realistic basis rather than for spite or to prove that she was right. Being right had been very important to her, since she was unwilling to admit any fault in the breakup of her marriage. The mistakes she made in the dance, and which she could not conceal, made it possible for her to admit it when she was wrong in other things. Her quarrelsome personality vanished, and she became a very attractive woman in both mind and body.

Student 2: Mrs. Y had, at one time, been very active in singing. After witnessing a terrible family tragedy in which her husband and child were killed, she suffered a breakdown from which she emerged in a highly nervous condition, and unable to produce melody or follow rhythm. During her course of psychiatric treatment, she started studying the dance because it looked like fun, and she thought it might take her mind off her troubles. At first, she was severely uncoordinated and approached the dance as a lark, making great fun of herself and her blunders. But she was exceptionally likable and vivacious, and other students quickly became her friends. When she saw that they took their dancing seriously and seemed to benefit by doing so, she stopped regarding herself as a clown. She had a costume made and studied the dance intensely, taking many classes and private lessons. She certainly never intended to dance professionally (money was of no concern; she donated scholarships to students who could not afford to pay), but she did enjoy performing at social functions sponsored by her church. Without her being aware of it, the dance served as a key to unlocking her problems with melody and rhythm, and also supplied a means of expression through which she could discard the clown mask and resume being herself.

There is no doubt that the dance helped these people, as it has helped many others. But we must remind ourselves again that the dance is not a panacea. On the other hand, there has never been a student, of the thousands who have studied belly dancing at Serena's studio, who has been harmed by it.

CHILDBIRTH

This has been singled out from the physical category because the presence, or absence, of it affects *all* women. For the sake of illustration and brevity, we have divided this section into three phases:

CONCEPTION

A number of women who had been trying for some time to become pregnant came to the studio to study the dance because they thought that perhaps the erotic nature of it might somehow enhance their fertility. The majority of them did conceive within a few months. Their doctors agree that the results are much more than mere chance, yet are at a loss to explain it. There were, however, several theories: *(1)* All but two of the women were overweight; some of them quite obese. It is possible that the weight loss unclogged the reproductive organs by removing constricting fat, or that the abdominal movements of the dance literally shook the lazy organs into activity. *(2)* They became more attractive to their husbands, who then tried harder. *(3)* Because of increased flexibility they cooperated more in the sex act.

PREGNANCY

One of Serena's students took private lessons well into her eighth month of pregnancy. She claims that she stopped because she became so large that it was difficult for her to do the steps, and her movements were awkward. Of course, she was a rare exception. She came to her lessons not only under the close supervision of her doctor, but in the company of her sister who is a physiotherapist. She is one of those women who believe firmly in natural childbirth, and she used the abdominal movements of the dance to strengthen the muscles which are called upon in delivery. Comparison of many of the steps outlined in this book with exercises suggested by proponents of natural childbirth will show a very close similarity. If you are interested in this application, consult your obstetrician.

Doctors agree that the old "cream puff" method of coddling the normal pregnant woman is a mistake. Treating pregnancy as an abnormality and greatly limiting physical activity can result in a variety of problems, one of which is varicose veins. Blood travelling back to the heart from the legs depends on valves in the veins and muscle action to transport it. The so-called *abdominal pump* supplies much of this action, and certainly the abdomen is a vital area to the dance.

POST PARTUM PERIOD

The time just following the birth of a child is usually a happy one for all concerned, though there are definite adjustments to be made. Some women are unable to make these adjustments easily and are disappointed to find that their new role as mother has resulted in the transfer of the attention which was once lavished on her to the baby. The levels of certain exhilarating hormones also drop suddenly after term in some women. One may then slip into what is often termed post partum depression, which is, very simply, a state of depression which follows giving birth. The dance often helps to overcome this depression by providing the new mother with a very personally rewarding activity, as well as giving her something to think about besides feeding the baby, washing the baby, cleaning up after the baby, etc. A woman is no more justified in neglecting herself than she is in neglecting her child.

The new mother is also often dismayed and depressed to find that her body doesn't have the glamorous shape it had before her pregnancy. Some women take one look at their stretch marks and flabby tummies and go on an eating jag in an attempt to drown their sorrows in food. Of course, the more they eat the worse they look, and the more sorry they feel for themselves . . . so they eat some more. The dance can help break this ugly cycle. It can keep weight down, tone the loose tummy, and restore her pride in herself. It's worth noting that exercising abdominal muscles has more than just cosmetic value: During pregnancy flabby muscles can stretch to the point where they actually part *(diastasis recti)*.

SEX

There is not a woman studying belly dancing who doesn't wonder what the dance will do to or for her sex life . . . especially if she doesn't have any! The answer is quite simple: The dance only helps to release the sensual and sexual *you* to its fullest capability. While it is true that the dance has been used for sexual instruction, the time for that need has long passed. There is absolutely nothing, including drugs, which will give you greater sexual pleasure, or make you a better lover than your nature allows. The secret of the belly dancer's sex appeal is her enthusiasm for sex.

Our attitude toward sex (publicly) covers a much broader range than it ever has before. Guilt is less of a problem because the moral climate is such that justification is easy to find for almost anything. But in our eagerness to get it all out in the open, the biological techniques have been stressed to the point where sex is being depersonalized. It is considered quaint to attach any significance to it other than as a pleasure mechanism, and this concept is just as restrictive as the rigid ethics it hopes to replace!

An interesting quotation, which examines our current styles of sexual thought and behavior, comes from a book by Widley Bradson:

"A peculiar introspection is taking place, so that the natural outpouring of sexual joy and fulfillment is turning on itself and freedom of expression for its own sake has become a misdirected pseudo-educated search for the impossible *supersex*.

"It's the eternal fable of the centipede: once he stops to wonder which of his hundred feet to put forward first, he so confuses himself that he is unable to walk at all. The simple, innocent enjoyment of sex is teetering in its own confusion. And at the core of it all are the great priapisms of our time, stirring the turbulence with their greedy ignorance . . . the petty voyeurs of psychology: *the sexperts*."

This is another way of saying that we give too much thought and planning to activities which are so natural that analyzing them only serves to confuse them and remove the romance, mystery, spontaneity . . . and of course, the *fun*. Sex can't be enjoyed according to rules or schedules, nor can it be appreciated to the impossible extent so juicily described by *sexperts*. Yet, it is surprising how many people are willing to suffer the bitter disappointments of their endless search for *supersex*.

Students have said that they have danced privately for their husbands, and admitted that they added a few special movements of their own. They found that the performance aroused both of them so much that the love-making which followed was intensely satisfying.

It is this healthy role-playing which adds variety to sex. And a trim, lithe body will enjoy greater participation than one that is stiff and unresponsive. You will discover that the remedies for stiffness and unresponsiveness are built into the steps; you won't have to think about them, or even look for them. The benefits will surprise you by simply being there when you want them most.

GETTING STARTED

This book is all you need to enjoy learning and exercising with the belly dance. The steps and movements are fully described and illustrated, and the tempos and rhythms are spelled out in words which you can recite to yourself as you go along. But if you are like Serena's students at her studio, you will want to have the fun of dancing and exercising to music. If you have any hope or desire to perform the dance before an audience, a musical background for your practice sessions is a *must,* since music is the framework on which the dance is based.

MUSIC

A phonograph is the best source of music. A wide variety of records is available, and you can easily play your favorite selections over and over (see Appendix I—Music). It is also possible to use a tape or cassette recorder, though it is difficult to locate the cuts you want. Another problem with tape is that there are very few taped recordings of Middle Eastern music on the market, so it will be necessary for you to copy recordings yourself wherever you can find them.

If you don't have a phonograph or tape recorder, you can use your radio. Of course you won't be able to select and repeat the songs you want, but music is a fundamental art, and you will find that moving to a variety of melodies and rhythms can be exciting and an enjoyable challenge. Also, if you live in a large city you will probably find foreign language stations which play authentic Middle Eastern music.

ATTIRE

Most of Serena's students wear leotards to class because they fit, as she says, "like a second skin." But it's not necessary to buy them if you don't already own them. Any clothing will do as well provided it is flexible, easy to move in, not bulky, and does not conceal the lines of your body. Some students prefer body-shirts, tank-type bathing suits, or bikinis. Heavier women often feel more comfortable in jersey shirts and slacks.

On her feet, Serena wears special dance shoes with a medium heel (as you can see in the illustrations). She admits that this is a departure from the naturalness of the dance. But as a professional performer she needs the support and protection they give her on all sorts of floor surfaces. She also agrees that heels give legs a more graceful taper. However, she suggests that women who are accustomed to wearing sandals or shoes without heels should wear soft dance slippers. Women who normally wear heels should wear low to medium heels with good support.

Do not attempt to dance in shoes whose heel height is different from that which you are used to wearing, as they will tend to throw you off balance. Serena will not allow her students to dance in spiked heels or shoes with pointed toes. Platform soles are also taboo because shoes must be extremely flexible to allow feet to move naturally.

OTHER ACCESSORIES

A mirror, full-length if available, can be very helpful in comparing your movements with Serena's as they appear in the illustrations. But if you practice in front of a mirror, be careful not to become dependent on it. If you get in the habit of dancing for your own reflection, you may find it very difficult to practice without it or to perform for an audience.

Some of the steps involve the use of a veil. For practice purposes your veil can be any piece of material, such as a bath towel, curtain, or an old sheet cut to approximately 72 by 45 inches.

Some students enjoy practicing in a dance skirt, which they feel makes them look better and gives them more to do. (For details on skirts, veils, and costumes see Appendix II—Costumes.)

You may have noticed professional dancers wearing small brass bells on their fingers. These bells are called *zills* and are played in time with the music. Serena never performs without them, but since they are of interest only to the student who expects to perform, they have been omitted from the regular lesson sections of the book. (For further information about zills, see Appendix I—Music.)

THE WARM-UP

You can't exercise unless you know the steps . . . and you can't do the steps properly unless you are in suitable physical condition. This is true at the outset of every practice session whether it's your first or hundred and first. Your body must be limbered and tuned to dance before you start. All athletes train to keep themselves in shape and dancers are no exception. They insist on a warm-up period before they play or perform, and they have an exercise routine they follow carefully.

The warm-up and conditioning exercises Serena has arranged for you consist of dance steps which will be used throughout the book. They have been selected because they are both excellent preparatory movements as well as being basic to the dance.

Once the warm-up steps have been learned along with Serena's special terms that apply to them, you will be able to create both your own dance and your own exercise system by combining movements of one part of the body with those of another . . . and even contrasting movements of the same part. The number of possible combinations of steps and movements is infinite, and it is up to each dancer to express her individuality and creative skill in evolving a dance which is uniquely hers. You should never be a slave to the steps. Instead, they should be the tools of your imagination.

Before you begin the warm-up steps which follow, a word of caution: Don't jump around in the book or attempt to progress too rapidly, and never overdo! Most of the warm-up steps are done *very slowly,* and you may be tempted to rush through them or repeat them too many times. Don't! The slow tempo is intended to develop coordination, control, and strength. It takes time to develop the power, stamina, and skill required to do the steps properly. Attempting advanced steps before you are ready for them can be discouraging and might be harmful.

And now, on with the dance!

Warm-up: Posture

Though not steps as such, posture and the two starting positions are as important to the dance as all of the movements combined. Poor posture makes it impossible to do the steps correctly, and at the same time lessens or destroys their exercise value.

The manner in which you carry yourself determines the mood and character of your dance. A proud woman does not slouch. Anything, including the human body, which is limp and sagging gives the impression of being sloppy, uninteresting, sluggish, and dull.

Your posture reflects your attitude toward life. Many otherwise intelligent people, in an effort to hang loose or look cool, assume an attitude of lazy indifference which is supposed to indicate their relaxed and confident outlook. Instead of seeming relaxed and assured, they often succeed in appearing unhinged and stupid. A drooping body is a poor substitute for poise in women who don't know what to do gracefully with their hands and feet; simply letting them hang, with hunched shoulders, alongside a limp body gives a whipped dog appearance.

There is also a posture which many women have

adopted because they think it is chic: the fashion model stance—shoulders forward, chest caved in, pelvis pushed forward, feet pigeon-toed. This may sell clothes from the pages of fashion magazines, but try and walk in that position!

There is more to posture than appearance. Compare the shape of your spine, in profile, to that of your pet dog or cat. You will notice that the animal's spine is straight, and that yours has an S shape. The reason for this is that the animal stands and walks on four legs and his spine is parallel to the ground. All of his internal organs are suspended from his spine. The S shape of your spine makes it possible for you to be comfortable in an upright position by distributing support where it is needed and evenly absorbing the strain. Obviously, poor posture results in an unnatural cramping of vital organs.

CORRECT POSTURE

Shoulders down, rib-cage elevated, back slightly arched, knees gently flexed, weight evenly distributed on both legs. This posture should require no effort, or produce strain. If you find that it does, you have been standing incorrectly.

Throughout your practice sessions be aware of your posture. But even more important, be aware of it during all your waking hours. You'll be surprised how people will notice.

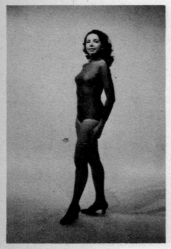

correct posture

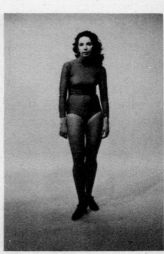

incorrect posture

Starting Positions

POSITION A
Place one foot in front of the other and turn both feet out slightly.

POSITION B
Place feet parallel to one another, about six inches apart; turn both feet out slightly.

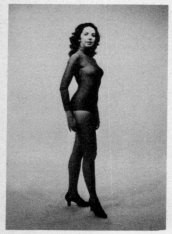

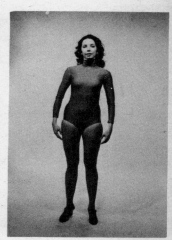

starting position A   *starting position B*

Serena's Warm-up Steps

STEP 1—SHOULDER SLIDE
Music: Slow (cifte telli)
ONE: Assume starting position A.
TWO: Slide shoulder to side being careful not to move hips or legs., Check in mirror to be sure that your shoulders are in a *straight line* and parallel to the floor.
NOTE: In order to get the straight line from shoulder to shoulder you will have to raise your shoulder slightly as you extend it. As women grow older, they have a tendency to become especially stiff through the shoulder area. If you experience this stiffness, you should attempt this movement gradually until maximum extension and stretch are achieved.
THREE: Straighten torso to starting position.
FOUR: Slide shoulders to the other side in a straight horizontal line as before; don't tilt or have one shoulder higher than the other.

FOR EXERCISE: Slide shoulders slowly to each side eight or more times.

Using the shoulder slide to learn the cifte telli rhythm:
ONE: Move shoulders to one side and say slowly out loud: ONE—PAUSE. . . .
TWO: Continuing, move shoulders smoothly to the other side, counting out loud: TWO—PAUSE. . . .
THREE: Move shoulders from side to side on remaining counts, one for each side: ONE—TWO—THREE.
FOUR: Repeat all the above, counting evenly. Allow the same amount of time for each word. (Also see Appendix I—Music, Cifte Telli.)
Since it takes longer to say "ONE—PAUSE" than it does

to say simply "ONE" by itself, we might think of this rhythm as: SLOW—SLOW—FAST—FAST—FAST, or in terms of shoulder movements RIGHT—PAUSE—LEFT—PAUSE—RIGHT—LEFT—RIGHT . . . continuing . . . LEFT—PAUSE—RIGHT—PAUSE—LEFT—RIGHT—LEFT.

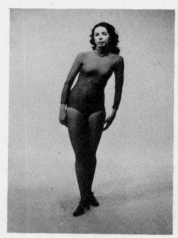

Step 1-2

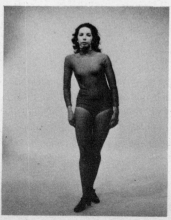

Step 1-4

STEP 2—SHOULDER SLANT

Music: Slow

ONE: Assume starting position A.

TWO: Slowly lower one shoulder toward hip on same side; at the same time raise other shoulder.

NOTE: Keep your arms loose and your hands relaxed. Do not tighten your fingers. Be careful with this, as with all movements, not to make unpleasant faces.

THREE: Lower the raised shoulder toward hip on the same side; at the same time, raise other shoulder.

FOR EXERCISE: Repeat at least eight times on each side.

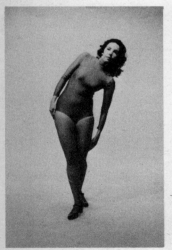 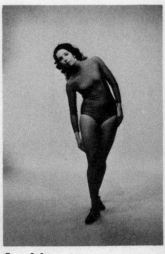

Step 2-2 *Step 2-3*

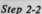

STEP 3—LARGE CIRCLE OF SHOULDERS

Music: Slow

ONE: Assume shoulder slide position (Step 1) with shoulders extended to one side.

TWO: Slowly arc shoulders to forward position; rib-cage and entire upper torso are forward.

THREE: Slide shoulders out to other side.

FOUR: Arc shoulders and upper torso around to the rear.

FIVE: Arc forward to starting position.

NOTE: During entire step, shoulders face forward and do not twist. Hips and legs do not move.

FOR EXERCISE: Do four shoulder circles in one direction, and then four in the opposite direction. For extra limbering, do four arcs in the forward position only, and four arcs in the rear position only.

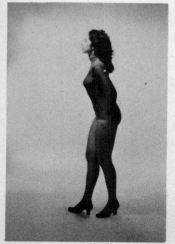

Step 3-2

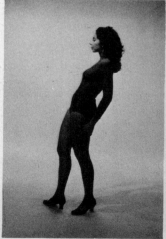

Step 3-4

STEP 4—SMALL SHOULDER CIRCLES

Music: Slow

ONE: Assume starting position A.

TWO: Bring one shoulder forward.

THREE: Raise shoulder *straight* up.

FOUR: With shoulder still in raised position, arc back as far as you can.

FIVE: With shoulder still in the back position, arc it downward.

SIX: Arc forward to starting position.

Variation: Starting with one shoulder in the forward *up* position and the other in the rear *down* position, rotate the shoulders simultaneously in the *same direction.* As they move, one shoulder will be arcing up while the other arcs down. This is an excellent exercise for coordination and control.

FOR EXERCISE: Repeat a minimum of eight times.

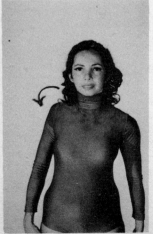

Step 4-4

STEP 5—SHOULDER THRUST
Music: Slow (rhumba)
ONE: Assume starting position A.
TWO: Thrust one shoulder forward: at the same time, thrust the other to the rear. Be careful not to move the rest of the body any more than necessary. Do not hunch!
THREE: Reverse movement, bringing forward shoulder to the rear; at the same time, bring rear shoulder forward.

Using the shoulder thrust to learn the rhumba rhythm:
Move your shoulders as above while saying aloud the following words LEFT—PAUSE—PAUSE—RIGHT—PAUSE—LEFT—PAUSE . . . RIGHT—PAUSE—PAUSE—LEFT—PAUSE—RIGHT—PAUSE.
Remember to give each word the same amount of time. (Also see Appendix I—Music, Rhumba.)

FOR EXERCISE: Do entire step eight times slowly, and eight times fast.

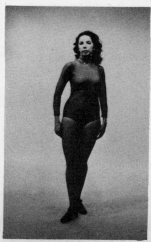

Step 5-2

STEP 6—RIB-CAGE EXTENSION

Music: Slow

ONE: Assume starting position A.

TWO: Bring rib-cage and shoulders forward, but do not bend at the waist. Your back should be arched.

THREE: Pull rib-cage in to posture shown; do not bend at the waist.

NOTE: Movement of one part of the body, excluding others, is called *isolation*. Isolating the rib-cage is difficult for most women because the movement is new to them and they are stiff. To be sure that you are doing this isolation correctly, place your fingertips against the lower "floating" rib on each side. You will not only feel the separation of torso elements as you move, but you will be able to guide your movement.

FOR EXERCISE: Repeat a minimum of eight times very slowly, and eight times quickly.

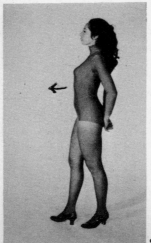

Step 6-2

STEP 7—RIB-CAGE CIRCLE

Music: Slow
ONE: Assume starting position A.
TWO: Move rib-cage to one side without twisting, tilting, or moving the lower part of your body.
THREE: Arc rib-cage forward.
FOUR: Continue arc to other side.
FIVE: Arc rib-cage to the rear.
SIX: Arc through to position 2 as above.

Variation: Do step as above, but move quickly through forward arc maintaining the rest of the movement at a slow pace; then repeat, speeding up the rear arc instead. This will have the effect of a fast accent in a basically slow series of movements.

FOR EXERCISE: Do four complete slow circles in one direction; four complete slow circles in the other. Repeat adding accents.

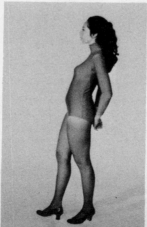

Step 7-5

STEP 8—SPINAL FLEX
Music: Slow

ONE: Assume starting position B.

TWO: Holding abdomen taut, move rib-cage forward. Without bending at waist or leaning back, **arch** your back as illustrated. If you are doing this movement properly, you will feel tension in the lower and upper back.

THREE: Bring shoulders and pelvis forward; pull rib-cage in. Throughout the remainder of the book, this position will be known as a **contraction.** Master this movement; it is important to the entire dance!

NOTE: This step can be done with varying degrees of arch and contraction. The beginning student should not attempt extremes, nor holding such positions for any length of time.

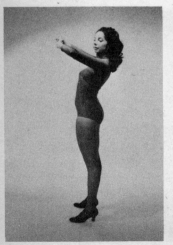

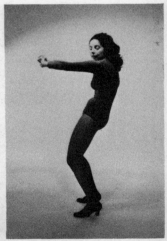

Step 8-2

Step 8-3

Exercise Variation: To firm chest muscles, bring shoulders *straight* down and flex chest muscles when in position 2 above.

FOR EXERCISE: Carefully, according to needs and ability.

STEP 9—HIP SLIDE
Music: Slow
ONE: Assume starting position B.
TWO: With both heels *remaining on the floor,* slide hip out to side as far as you can so that your weight is on the leg of the extended hip. Keep both knees *slightly* bent; do not let either knee buckle! Check to see that your right shoulder is directly over your right foot and that your left shoulder is directly over your left foot.
THREE: Return to starting position B.
FOUR: Slide hip out to other side in same manner as 2 above.

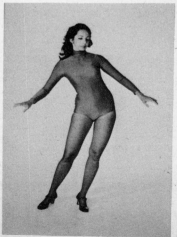

Step 9-2

Variations: 1. With hip extended, bear down on the leg holding your weight and snap hip to other side. Done correctly, this is an excellent toning exercise for the entire mid-section.

2. Begin with hips extended to one side, in hip slide position, knees slightly bent. Slowly bend both knees; lower torso and arc hips down, but keep body straight. Arc hips out to the other side; *straighten knees,* and hold extended hip slide position.

NOTE: As you bend knees, do not push derrière to rear. This step is excellent for firming thighs.

FOR EXERCISE: Repeat, with variations, a minimum of ten times.

STEP 10—HIP SWIVEL
Music: Slow

ONE: Assume starting position B, with arms extended out at sides as illustrated.

TWO: Tense muscle of right upper-arm. When done correctly, this muscle will contract and appear to swell while the rest of the arm remains loose. Master this isolated tension now, as it will appear as an important part of more advanced movements. Push right arm back slightly, forcing *right* hip to arc forward. Do not move your feet. Hips should be turned slightly to the side; shoulders remain facing forward.

THREE: Tense muscles in left upper-arm. Arc left hip forward as right hip arcs back.

NOTE: Try to have as little movement in your arms as possible. Check in your mirror to see that your arms have a relaxed look even though they are tense. Obvious tension results in a grotesque Frankenstein's Monster appearance. Seeming to be relaxed when in a state of tension is an important fundamental in both dance and exercise.

FOR EXERCISE: Repeat eight times slowly, and eight times quickly.

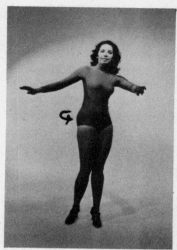

Step 10-2

STEP 11—PELVIC TILT
Music: Slow
ONE: Assume starting position B.
TWO: Tense muscles of mid-section, buttocks, and thighs. Bend knees, at the same time, lower and tilt pelvis upward. When you are in the proper position, your body will be in a straight line from knees to shoulders.

FOR EXERCISE: Hold pelvic tilt position for a slow count of twenty.

Combination Exercise: Combine Step 11 (pelvic tilt) with Step 5 (shoulder thrust). Be aware of the muscle groups you are using, and of the coordination involved. Check in your mirror to be sure that your movements are never jerky or sudden.

FOR EXERCISE: Hold pelvic tilt position for a slow count of twenty; at the same time, add ten shoulder thrusts.

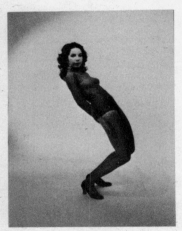

Step 11-2

STEP 12—KNEE DIP AND TWIST
Music: Medium rhumba
ONE: Assume starting position B.
TWO: (Attempt this movement carefully at first!) Bend knees, turning hips slightly to the side. Do not move feet; be sure to bend *both* knees.
THREE: Straighten to starting position.
FOUR: Bend knees as above to other side.

FOR EXERCISE: Eight times on right side; eight times on left side. Then alternate eight times.

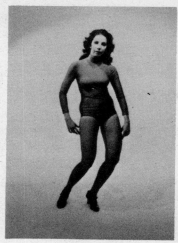

Step 12-2

STEP 13—KNEELING SIT-UP
Music: Slow

ONE: Assume kneeling position as shown; knees about four inches apart. Do not crumple in the mid-section. Keep your back slightly arched.

TWO: Sit down *very* slowly until you are resting on your calves.

THREE: Raise very slowly to kneeling position. Properly done, this movement will cause tension in your thighs.

FOR EXERCISE: Do slowly twelve times.

Combination: Combine kneeling sit-up with shoulder slide (Step 1).

FOR EXERCISE: According to your needs and ability. Don't overdo!

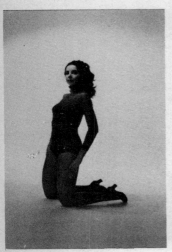

Step 13-1   *Step 13-2*

STEP 14—KNEE-BEND WITH ARCHED BACK
Music: Slow
ONE: Assume arched spine position as in spinal flex (Step 8).
TWO: Slowly bend knees forward, maintaining arch. Keep your heels on the floor!
THREE: Slowly return to starting position.

Variation: Try deeper knee-bend with heels raised off the floor.

FOR EXERCISE: Do step (with or without variation)

eight times slowly. Do not vary the arch. Hold bend a
few seconds before rising.

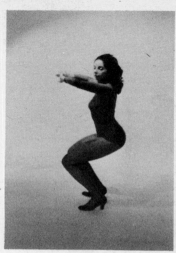

Step 14-2

STEP 15—KNEE-BEND HOLDING CONTRACTION

Music: Slow

ONE: Assume contracted position as in part 2 of spinal
flex (Step 8).

TWO: Slowly bend your knees maintaining contracted
position. Keep your heels on the floor!

THREE: Return to starting position.

Variation: Move as above, but into a deeper knee-bend
and with heels raised from floor.

FOR EXERCISE: Repeat eight times, holding bend for
a few seconds each time.

Combination: Hold bend, and in this position do spinal flex (Step 8). Your torso position changes from arch to contraction and back again. You will feel tension in the calves of your legs and will find this movement to be quite strenuous.

FOR EXERCISE: According to needs and ability, but use caution!

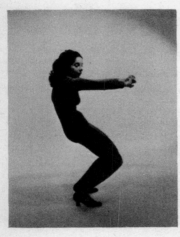

Step 15-2

STEP 16—HEEL BOUNCE
Music: Slow (cifte telli, rhumba) or fast
ONE: Assume starting position B.
TWO: Raise both heels rapidly off floor about one inch. At peak proceed smoothly; do not hold the lifted heel position.
THREE: Quickly lower heels to floor.
NOTE: Practice counting rhythm with this step as follows:

2/4 Rhythm (See Appendix I—Music)

ONE	TWO	ONE	TWO
Up down	up	down	up

Raise heels and come down on the count of ONE. Count evenly and say the words aloud. Stay in the down position until you have said the word TWO (don't move on the word itself), and raise into the up position so that you can come down again on the count of ONE. Also practice this step with the cifte telli and the rhumba.

FOR EXERCISE: This is great exercise for the calves and legs if done to the point where you can *just* feel the tension. As with all exercises, do not test your endurance!

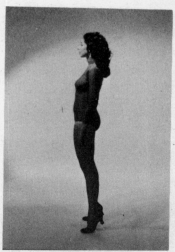

Step 16-2

BEGINNER STEPS

STEP 17—ARM CIRCLE
BODY TYPES: 3, 5
Exercise: Shoulders, upper-arms
Music: Slow
ONE: Assume starting position A, arms at sides, palms
in.
TWO: Slowly lift arms out at sides, palms facing down,
elbows gently curved.

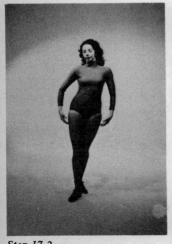

Step 17-2

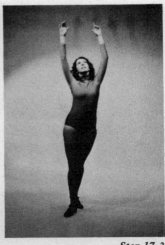

Step 17-3

THREE: As you stretch your arms up over your head, turn wrists so palms face each other. Stretch high, but keep shoulders down.

FOUR: Cross wrists with palms facing to rear. Lower arms in front of you, palms facing you, to starting position.

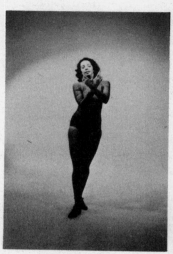

Step 17-4

Variation: To add faster accent, lower arms slowly; when they reach chest level, drop them quickly to starting position; then continue slowly to repeat. The building of tension, with a controlled release is a natural life-cycle, which is the basis of dramatic action. Keep this in mind while learning all steps.

Combination: As you raise arms above head, slowly arch spine as in spinal flex (Step 8); as you lower your arms in front of you, contract torso as in spinal flex (Step 8).

STEP 18—PARALLEL ARM CIRCLE

BODY TYPES: 3, 5, 6
Exercise: Arms, shoulders, chest, upper back
Music: Slow

ONE: Assume starting position A.

TWO: Stretch arms above head, palms facing each other.

THREE: Bend to position illustrated.

FOUR: Turn palms downward as you lower arms at side.

FIVE: Bring arms down in front of you; bend knees slightly and contract torso as in spinal flex (Step 8).

SIX: As you raise arms to other side, turn palms down.

SEVEN: Stretch arms out on other side as illustrated.

EIGHT: Return to starting position.

NOTE: Arms move in a circular pattern like the hands of clocks. To draw attention to your movements, follow them with your head and eyes.

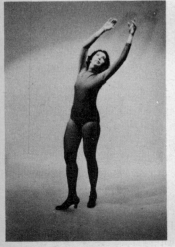

Step 18-3   *Step 18-4*

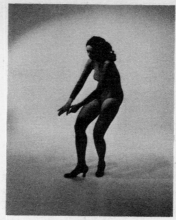

Step 18-5

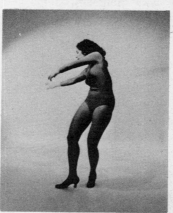

Step 18-7

Variation: For faster accent, do step slowly until you reach position 3; move quickly to position 7 and continue slowly. This is another example of tension created by very slow movement, and complete release by muscle relaxation. Serena has developed this to a high degree and uses it extensively.

STEP 19—KNEELING PARALLEL ARM CIRCLE

BODY TYPES: 3, 5, 6
Exercise: Shoulders, thighs, mid-section
Music: Slow (cifte telli)

ONE: Assume kneeling position as in kneeling sit-up (Step 13).

TWO: Stretch arms above your head, palms facing each other.

THREE: Slowly lower arms out at sides, palms down, as illustrated. Shoulders slant as in shoulder slant (Step 12).

FOUR: Bring shoulders forward; brush arms lightly across floor; contract torso.

FIVE: Lift arms to position illustrated; slowly turn palms to face down.

SIX: Lift arms with shoulders slanted as illustrated.

SEVEN: Return to starting position.

NOTE: Many kneeling steps, including this one, were created by Berber women who, because of their low tents, were forced to dance on their knees!

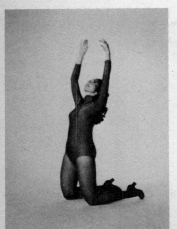

Step 19-2

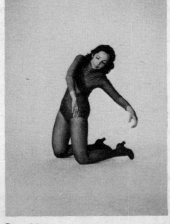

Step 19-3

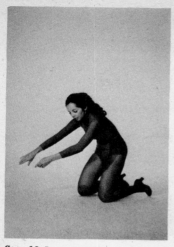 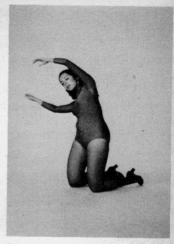

Step 19-5 *Step 19-6*

Variations: 1. Reverse the circle and move in the opposite direction; add faster accent by moving quickly from position 3 to position 5.

2. On upward stretch of arms, push shoulders back with large arch of spine. As arms come forward, sit back on calves, exaggerate torso contraction until angle of spine is parallel to floor.

3. Occasionally omit stretch of arms (position 2) and repeat forward sweep of arms from one side to the other, then continue to position 2.

4. Move to cifte telli rhythm as follows: (a) Starting from any arm position in circle, move arms one-quarter of the way around (*i.e.,* from 12 o'clock to 3 o'clock) on the counts: ONE—PAUSE—TWO—PAUSE. (b) Swing arms to opposite side and back (*i.e.,* 3 o'clock to 9 o'clock) moving as hands of clock, on counts: ONE—TWO—THREE. If you start at 12 o'clock, you will finish at 9 o'clock.

STEP 20—FIGURE 8 OF HANDS

BODY TYPES: All
Exercise: Especially good for older women in toning skin of hands
Music: Slow

ONE: Assume starting position A.

TWO: With arms loose at sides, turn wrists so that palms face to the rear.

THREE: Move arms and hands slowly forward at hip level, bending wrists to face each other. Palms now face to sides.

FOUR: Move wrists toward each other until they are four inches apart. Palms still face to side.

FIVE: Turns wrists so that palms face each other.

SIX: Arc wrists back, palms forward, brushing hips with edge of palms.

SEVEN: When hands are three inches behind hips, slowly turn wrists so that palms face to the rear.

EIGHT: Bring arms forward to starting position.

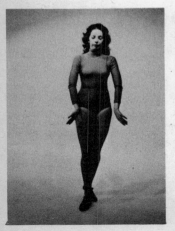

Step 20-2

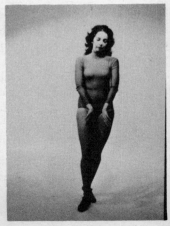

Step 20-4

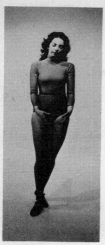
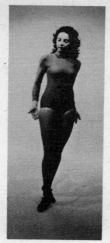
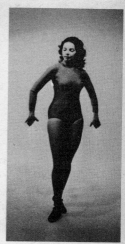

Step 20-5   *Step 20-6*   *Step 20-7*

NOTE: Keep fingers relaxed; hands must look graceful. Do not separate fingers and tense them, as this will result in ugly witches' claws.

Variation: Start with hands raised at various levels of arm circle (Step 17).

Combinations: 1. Combine with spinal flex (Step 8). As you bring your arms forward, contract torso; as you move your arms behind you, arch your spine.
2. Combine with kneeling sit-up (Step 13).
3. Combine with pelvic tilt (Step 11).

STEP 21—ALTERNATING FIGURE 8 OF HANDS WITH THORAX TWIST

BODY TYPES: All

Exercise: Waist through upper torso

Music: Slow

NOTE: Before starting this step, practice Step 19 using each arm individually.

ONE: Assume starting position A.

TWO: Bring one arm forward, palm facing to the rear; at the same time, bring shoulder on same side forward so that upper torso twists to side and other arm is behind hip, palm facing forward.

THREE: Turn wrist of forward arm so that palm faces up and slightly away from you; at the same time, turn wrist of arm that is behind you so that palm faces to the rear.

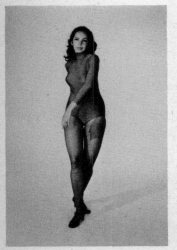

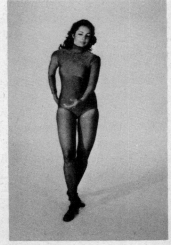

Step 21-2   *Step 21-3*

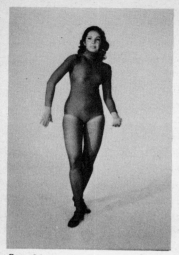

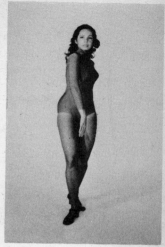

Step 21-4   *Step 21-5*

FOUR: Without changing curve of either arm, turn entire thorax so that rear shoulder and arm move forward, as front shoulder and arm move back to position illustrated. FIVE: Turn wrists and change direction of arms and shoulders, moving as in part 2 above.

NOTE: Hips face forward throughout step. If done correctly you will feel a pull through the waistline.

Combination: Combine with kneeling sit-up (Step 13).

STEP 22—TURKISH ARM POSE

BODY TYPES: 3, 6
Exercise: Shoulders, upper-arms (isometric)
Music: Any; used with all rhythms and tempos

ONE: Assume starting position A.

TWO: Slowly raise arms above head as in arm circle (Step 17), palms facing each other a few inches apart. Keep your shoulders down!

THREE: Cross wrists as illustrated.

FOUR: Turn wrists so that palms face each other.

FIVE: Press palms together as illustrated. Arms should be directly over your head.

NOTE: Simple as it looks, this step is easy to fumble. Practice it until you can do it smoothly.

Combinations: 1. Combine with the rib-cage circle (Step 7).

2. Combine with the spinal flex (Step 8).

3. Combine with the kneeling sit-up (Step 13).

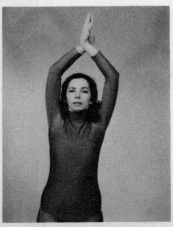

Step 22-5

STEP 23—HIP EXTENSION

BODY TYPE: 4

Exercise: Hips, thighs

Music: Any; used with all rhythms and tempos

ONE: Assume starting position B.

TWO: Raise hip by lifting heel from floor; do not bend knee. Slide shoulders (as in shoulder slide, Step 1) away from extended hip. Weight should be on leg opposite extended hip.

THREE: Repeat on other side.

NOTE: Study the difference between the hip extension and the hip slide (Step 9). Notice that in the hip slide, *your weight is on the leg of the extended hip.* Also, the angle of the legs is entirely different. This movement is important to many advanced steps, and will be referred to often.

Combination: Combine with Turkish arm pose (Step 22).

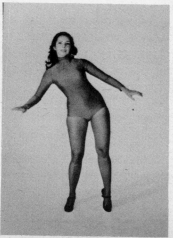

Step 23-2

STEP 24—HEAD SLIDE AND HEAD CIRCLE
BODY TYPES: All
Exercise: Head and neck; excellent for double chins
Music: Any; used with all rhythms and tempos
ONE: Assume starting position A.
TWO: Face forward. Do not turn, tilt, or slant head in any way. Move head to one side using neck muscles.
THREE: Return to starting position.
FOUR: Extend head to the other side.

NOTE: Your head should slide from side to side in a straight line as though floating on your shoulders.

Combinations: 1. Combine with Turkish arm pose (Step 22). Hold arms still as you move your head!
2. Combine with kneeling sit-up (Step 13).

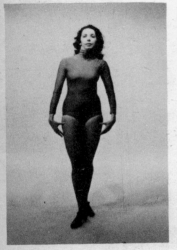
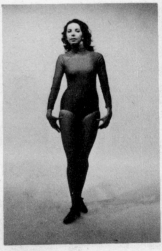

Step 24-2

Step 24-4

Variation: The head circle.

ONE: Stretch head and neck straight back as illustrated.
TWO: Arc through head slide position 2 to forward position as illustrated.
THREE: Arc through head slide position 4 to rear position as illustrated.

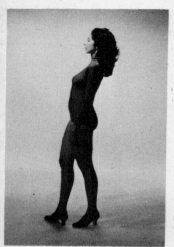

Step 24 var.-1

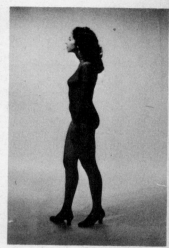

Step 24 var.-3

Combination: Combine with Turkish arm pose (Step 22).

Variation: There is an African step in which the head is moved in a circle as though the nose were tracing a large circle printed on a wall before it. The movement is usually done rather quickly, resulting in a wild appearance. Serena does not use this step, but many dancers do, and it is worthwhile learning, especially for the exercise value.

STEP 25—HIP CIRCLE

BODY TYPES: 2, 4

Exercise: Hips, waist

Music: Slow, fast

ONE: Assume starting position B, arms out at sides; slide hips all the way to the left as in hip slide position (Step 9), knees almost straight.

TWO: Slowly arc hips forward; bend knees slightly; pull shoulders back.

THREE: Continue arcing hips to the right; at the same time, straighten knees.

FOUR: Continue arcing hips to the rear; at the same time, bring shoulders forward, arching spine slightly. At this point knees should be very straight.

FIVE: Arc hips all the way to left side in hip slide position, knees almost straight.

Variations: 1. Move much more quickly on forward arc of hips; much more slowly on rear arc.

2. Move slowly on forward arc of hips, much faster on rear arc.

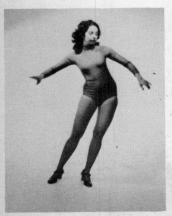

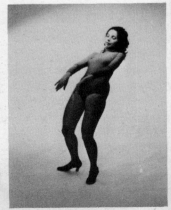

Step 25-1   *Step 25-2*

Combinations: 1. Combine with slow figure 8 of hands (Step 20). On forward arc of hips, hands face front; on rear arc of hips, hands are behind hip three to four inches. Keep hands at hip level throughout.
2. To dance with faster rhythms, combine with heel bounce (Step 16).

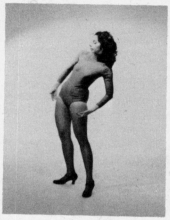

Step 25-3

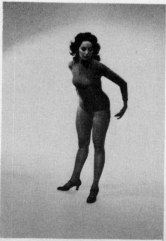

Step 25-4

STEP 26—FORWARD DIP AND CONTRACTION

BODY TYPES: 2, 4, 5
Exercise: Great for the waist!
Music: Bright 4/4

ONE: Assume starting position A.

TWO: Bend knees forward and contract torso. (Degree of bend can vary.)

THREE: Snap knees straight as you bring your shoulders to an exaggerated forward position.

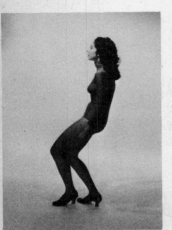

Step 26-2   *Step 26-3*

NOTE: To count 4/4 rhythm:

ONE	TWO	THREE	FOUR
Bend	Hold	Snap	Hold

For faster tempos, start with knees bent:

ONE	TWO	THREE	FOUR
Snap	Bend	Snap	Bend

STEP 27—STEP—POINT—STEP

BODY TYPES: 2, 4, 5

Exercise: Good for coordination

Music: Slow and fast

ONE: Assume starting position B with feet about three inches apart, arms raised at sides.

TWO: Lift right foot one inch off floor.

THREE: Lower right foot to floor; hold briefly.

FOUR: Extend left hip, lifting left heel and sliding left foot out to side about twelve inches; rest toe lightly on floor as though pointing. Stretch shoulders to right; hold briefly.

FIVE: Lower left foot to floor; hold briefly.

SIX: Extend right hip, lifting right heel and sliding right foot out to side about twelve inches and rest toe lightly on floor as though pointing. Stretch shoulders to left; hold briefly.

NOTE: This is an extremely important step and is used as a basis for both fast and slow dance segments.

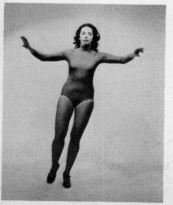

Step 27-2

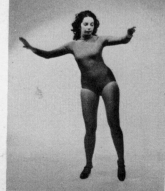

Step 27-4

Variations: 1. Turn torso toward extended hip on each extension.

2. To travel using this step, instead of stepping straight down, step forward (or back) a few inches.

Combinations: 1. Add subtle knee-bends to accent *fast* rhythms. This will give a happy bounce to your movements.

2. Combine with the arm circle (Step 17).

3. Combine with the figure 8 of hands (Step 20).

NOTE: When combining the step—point—step with arm patterns, *the arms move slowly even when the music is fast.* On some bright rhythms, it may take as many as six complete step—point—steps to allow enough time to do one complete slow arm circle or one complete figure 8 of hands. If you rush the arm movements, you will create a windmill appearance which is *never* correct and always looks awkward.

To count faster (brighter) rhythms with the step—point —step:

ONE	TWO	THREE	FOUR
Step down	Pause	Point	Pause

To count slower rhythms with the step—point—step:

ONE	PAUSE	TWO	PAUSE
Step	Hold	Point	Hold

ONE	TWO	THREE	PAUSE
Step	Hold	Point	Hold

Slide or drag to point instead of lifting your feet.

STEP 28—VEIL ARM CIRCLE
(Standing and Kneeling)

BODY TYPES: All

Exercise: Excellent for grace and coordination

Music: Slow (rhumba, cifte telli)

ONE: Assume starting position A. Hold veil by thumb and index fingers of each hand, about 36 inches apart, as illustrated.

TWO: Arc right arm forward; at the same time, twist upper torso to the left.

THREE: Arc right arm over your head so that elbow is directly over your right ear; arch your spine.

FOUR: Hold the veil directly behind your head as illustrated.

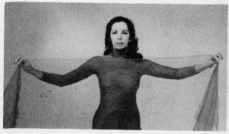

Step 28-1

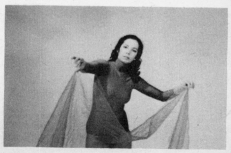

Step 28-2

FIVE: Tilt to the right as illustrated. Left hand should be directly over right hand by about fourteen inches.

SIX: Hold right hand still and in position; arc left hand to starting position.

Variation: Assume kneeling position as illustrated. Move your arms as for standing veil circle. Notice that your torso has a more exaggerated tilt than in standing position.

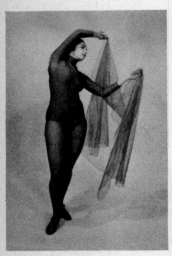

Step 28-3

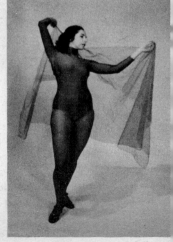

Step 28-4

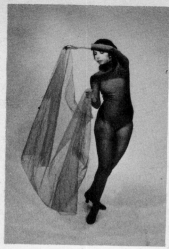

Step 28-5

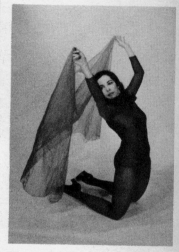

Step 28 var.-kneeling

Adding Accents: Add flowing, rapid movements on either forward or backward position of step.

NOTE: Master the positions where the veil is held directly in front of or behind torso. You will later combine other steps with these two positions to complete your veil dance. Serena has included veil movements in her suggested routines, although you are encouraged to create your own. When used properly, the veil becomes an extension of your body rather than just a prop or piece of fabric.

STEP 29—BASIC WALK

BODY TYPES: 2, 4, 5
Exercise: Legs, thighs; stamina, grace
Music: Medium to bright·

ONE: Assume starting position B, feet two inches apart.

TWO: Lift your right heel three inches off the floor as you bend both knees as illustrated.

THREE: Step forward three inches with right foot as both knees straighten.

FOUR: Lift left heel three inches off floor as you bend both knees.

FIVE: Step forward three inches with left foot as both knees straighten.

Variation: Use *very* small knee-bends with a much faster walk.

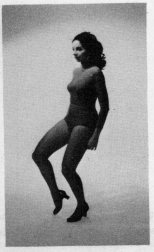

Step 29-2

Counting rhythm with the basic walk: 4/4

ONE	TWO	THREE	FOUR
Step	Bend	Step	Bend

Combinations: 1. Combine with arm circle (Step 17).
2. Combine with figure 8 of hands (Step 20).

NOTE: Keep arm patterns slow! You will do several steps before completing one entire arm movement!
3. Combine with spinal flex (Step 8) in this manner: Contract when you bend your knees; arch spine when you straighten knees.

STEP 29A—BASIC GLIDING WALK
BODY TYPES: 2, 4, 5
Exercise: Balance, poise
Music: Slow
ONE: Assume starting position A, right foot in front, knees slightly bent, arms out at sides.
TWO: Lift left heel one-half inch from floor; slide ball of left foot, in arcing pattern twelve inches to the left, and forward to a position twelve inches directly in front of right foot.
THREE: Lift right heel one-half inch from floor; slide ball of right foot, in arcing pattern twelve inches to the right, and forward to a position twelve inches directly in front of left foot.
FOUR: Repeat from part 2 above.

NOTE: As you glide forward, keep torso erect in gently arched spine position; move without raising or lowering torso.

Variations: 1. Repeat step, moving to the rear.

2. Bend knees more deeply and hold throughout. (Great exercise for thighs!)

Combinations: 1. Combine with arm circle (Step 17).
2. Combine with figure 8 of hands (Step 20).
3. Combine with alternating figure 8 of hands with thorax twist (Step 21).
4. Combine with Turkish arm pose (Step 22).

STEP 30—KNEE SLIDE
BODY TYPES: 2, 4, 5
Exercise: Especially good for the thighs
Music: Slow (cifte telli, rhumba)
ONE: Kneeling as in Step 13; arms out at sides.
TWO: Sit down slowly, moving right knee to the right twelve inches.
THREE: Slide left knee alongside right knee as you raise torso back to kneeling position.

Combination: (Difficult!) Combine with kneeling parallel arm circle (Step 19).

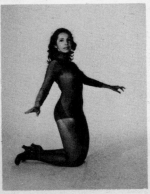

Step 30-1

STEP 31—FINGER RIPPLE

BODY TYPES: All
Exercise: Especially good for older women
Music: Any; all rhythms and tempos
ONE: Assume any starting position.
TWO: With hands in front of you, straighten fingers and curve them as shown in illustration.
THREE: Bend wrists, bringing fingertips down. Do not move your arms or change the curve of your fingers.
FOUR: Cup fingers as if holding an orange in each hand. Do not make claws.
FIVE: Hold finger positions, and arc wrists toward each other until palms face upward.
SIX: Slowly uncurl fingers, starting at base.
SEVEN: Very gradually, unfold fingers to straighten.

NOTE: Repeat movement until fingers ripple smoothly.

Variation: As you continuously ripple fingers, turn hands slowly so that palms face away from you, then turn hands back to starting position.

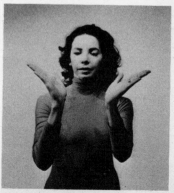

Step 31-2

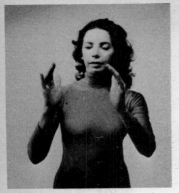
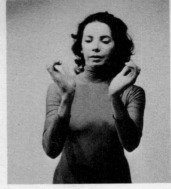

Step 31-3   *Step 31-6*

Combinations: 1. Combine variation with arm circle (Step 17).

2. Try creating your own arm movements and combine them with the finger ripple. Hands may be moved any distance apart.

BEGINNER ROUTINE 1 (SLOW)

ONE: Assume starting position A.

TWO: Do one slow arm circle (Step 17).

THREE: Repeat slow arm circle once, and combine with spinal flex (Step 8).

FOUR: Go smoothly into figure 8 of hands (Step 20) and do once.

FIVE: Add spinal flex to figure 8 of hands, and do once.

SIX: Slide feet into starting position B.

SEVEN: Do slow hip circle combined with figure 8 of hands, once in each direction.

EIGHT: Go smoothly into combination of slow step—point—step (Step 27) and arm circle; do four times forward, and four times backward.

NINE: Go back to starting position A.

TEN: Do slow figure 8 of hands; repeat twice.

ELEVEN: Merge into alternating figure 8 of hands with thorax twist (Step 21); repeat twice.

TWELVE: Slowly bring arms up to Turkish arm pose (Step 22); hold pose and do head slide (Step 24) to finish.

BEGINNER ROUTINE 2 (BRIGHT)

ONE: Assume starting position A.

TWO: Travel around edge of room with basic walk (Step 29) with arms out at sides.

THREE: When back at starting point, go into combination of step—point—step (Step 27) and slow figure 8 of hands (Step 20); repeat eight times forward and eight times back.

FOUR: Do variation 1 of the step—point—step, in place; twice on each side.

FIVE: Do forward dip and contraction (Step 26); repeat six times.

SIX: Do combination of hip circle (Step 25) and heel bounce variation (Step 16); repeat once in each direction.

SEVEN: Go back to combination of basic walk and arm circle; go forward eight steps, backward eight steps.

NOTE: Smile more during fast movements; be more thoughtful during slow movements. Watch arms and hands for angularity and jerkiness.

INTERMEDIATE STEPS

Introduction to Intermediate Steps

From this point on, your dancing will take on greater meaning as you become more familiar with the steps and as you create your own. You will notice that you will spend less time being concerned about exercise as such, and that you will be able to do more strenuous movements for a greater length of time.

As you progress through this section, you will see that there are special combination challenge steps at the end of each lesson. They are intended to "keep you on your toes" and to inspire the serious dancer. But they are also excellent exercise, and I suggest that everyone try them if only for the stimulating fun that comes from confronting a new and difficult problem.

Now that you will be attempting more complex steps, as well as intricate combinations, you should begin to consider what Serena calls *step families*. That is, you should become aware of points of similarity among the steps because these are the points at which transitions are the easiest and the most natural. It is by grouping these step families and their transitions that you will evolve your own dances.

CAUTION: Some of the steps in this and succeeding sections are difficult and strenuous. Do not disregard the warnings and advice given with these steps. Do not push yourself or practice when you feel fatigued. Do not attempt to advance more rapidly than your body will allow, and use a chair or other solid object for support when practicing steps requiring great balance or coordination. Remember, stamina and strength are achieved by exercising to a point *just beyond* that to which you are accustomed, and then resting sufficiently to allow your body to build to the new level.

STEP 32—PIVOT BOUNCE
BODY TYPES: 3, 4, 6
Exercise: Thighs, lower back, mid-section
Music: Bright 4/4 (also, 9/8)
NOTE: Refer to forward dip and contraction (Step 26), and perfect it before starting this step.
ONE: Assume starting position A.
TWO: Lift rear heel from floor; raise and stretch your arms in front of your body as illustrated.
THREE: Bend knees in contracted torso position.
FOUR: Push buttocks back, and move upper torso forward; at the same time, straighten both legs, turning about

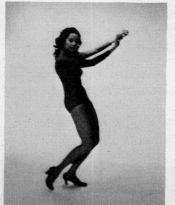
Step 32-3

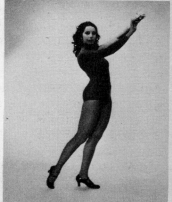
Step 32-4

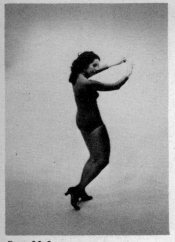

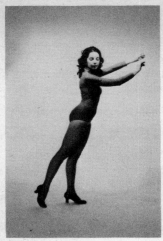

Step 32-5   *Step 32-6*

one-sixth of circle. (If right leg is in front, turn to the right; reverse if left leg is in front.)

FIVE: Bend both knees and contract again.

SIX: Straighten knees, arching spine as in part 4 above.

NOTE: It should take six complete knee-bends to complete a full circle. Be sure to practice this step turning in opposite direction, too.

To count with 4/4 rhythm: Start with knees straight.

ONE	TWO	THREE	FOUR
Bend	Hold	Straighten	Hold

To count with fast 4/4 rhythm: Start with knees bent.

ONE	TWO	THREE	FOUR
Straighten	Bend	Straighten	Bend

STEP 33—SNAKE ARMS
BODY TYPES: 3, 5, 6
Exercise: Shoulders and upper-arms
Music: Slow

NOTE: This step is difficult, but it is one of the prettiest of all arm movements. It is used often and should be perfected.

ONE: Assume starting position A. Bend elbows slightly, arms down at sides, palms in as illustrated.

TWO: Turn left shoulder in slightly and to the front.

THREE: Holding arm curve, raise left arm as high as you can as though a string were attached to your elbow and pulling upward. Palm should face in toward you, and your entire arm should make a C curve facing down. Check angle of arm in mirror.

FOUR: Raise hand so that it is parallel to your body, as illustrated. Look straight ahead, and do not twist body. In raising your hand, your elbow will turn down and your

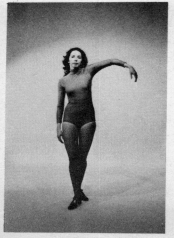

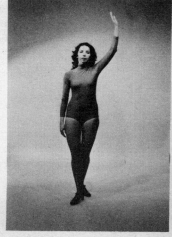

Step 33-3   Step 33-4

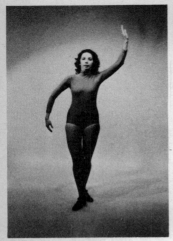

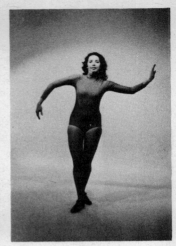

Step 33-5　　　　　　　　　　*Step 33-6*

forearm will rise. With your elbow at chin level, your entire arm will make a C curve facing up.

FIVE: Turn right shoulder in slightly and to the front. Right arm will be in position illustrated. At the same time, lower left arm with elbow facing down as illustrated.

SIX: Check this *halfway point:* Your arms should curve (as in picture) in the shape of an S.

SEVEN: Without changing arm position, continue raising right arm and lowering left arm.

EIGHT: Lower your right arm with elbow facing down as you turn the shoulder of your left arm and raise your left arm with elbow facing up.

NINE: Continue opposing movements maintaining S curve of arms.

Variation: For a faster, or rippling, effect keep up-and-down movement limited so that elbows travel only about twelve inches.

Combinations: 1. Combine with the shoulder slide (Step 1). As you lift right arm, slide right shoulder to the right. This is excellent exercise!

2. Combine with the kneeling sit-up (Step 13).

3. *Challenge combination:* Combine with the shoulder slide (Step 1), while holding your body in pelvic tilt position (Step 11).

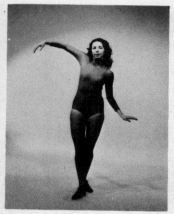

Step 33-7

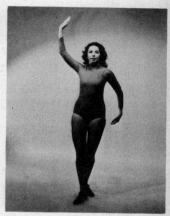

Step 33-8

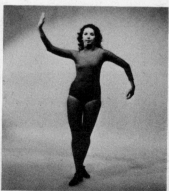

Step 33-9

STEP 34—CLASSIC ARMS

BODY TYPES: 3, 5, 6
Exercise: Shoulders and upper-arms.
Music: Slow

ONE: Assume starting position A.

TWO: Stretch your right arm high over your head, palm facing forward. Turn left palm to face rear, turning left shoulder in slightly.

THREE: Slowly lower extended right arm with palm facing forward, fingers up, elbow facing down. At the same time, raise left arm, palm facing to rear, fingers down.

FOUR: Continue above movements with arms passing each other in front of you at chest level. Don't change wrist angle!

FIVE: Lower right arm all the way; at the same time, lift your left arm high over your head.

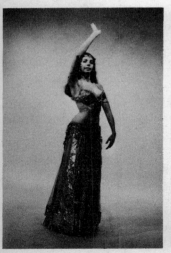

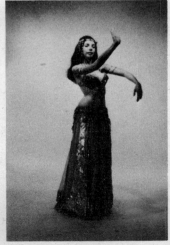

Step 34-2   *Step 34-3*

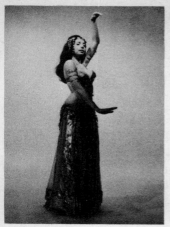

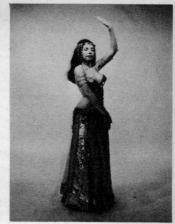

Step 34-5   *Step 34-6*

SIX: Hold these arm positions for a moment. Bend your
left wrist to point fingertips upward with palm facing out.
Point fingertips of right hand down with palm facing to
the rear.
SEVEN: Lift your right arm with palm facing to the rear;
lower left arm with palm facing forward.

Remember: When either arm is being raised, the palm
always faces down and to the rear; when either arm is
being lowered, the palm faces up and to the front.

Variation: For a faster, or rippling, effect move arms at
chest level no more than eight inches apart.

Combinations: 1. Combine with pelvic tilt (Step 11).
2. Combine with kneeling sit-up (Step 13).
3. *Challenge combination:* Use this step as you ripple
   fingers (Step 31), and move torso in slow spinal flex
   (Step 8).

STEP 35—HINDOO ARM STEP

BODY TYPES: All
Exercise: Arms, back, thighs
Music: Rhumba.

ONE: Assume starting position B. Place your weight on your left leg.

TWO: Raise both arms in front of you to chest level, elbows curved, palms facing in toward you. Step to the right about twelve inches with your right foot. Shift your weight to your right leg, and hold for a moment.

THREE: Slowly lift your right arm above your head; move your left arm out to the left parallel to the floor; lift left heel.

FOUR: With left heel up, slide ball of left foot behind right foot about twelve inches; at the same time, tilt upper torso to the right and bend both knees as illustrated. Hold pose and look up at right arm.

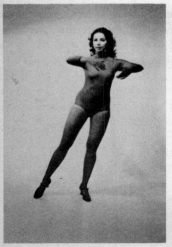

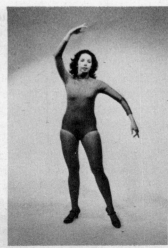

Step 35-2   *Step 35-3*

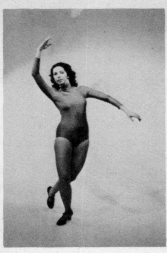

Step 35-4

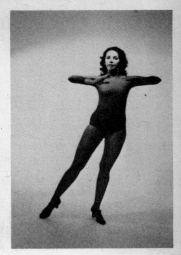

Step 35-5

FIVE: Slide left foot eighteen inches to left of right foot. Slowly bring hands together so that fingertips are about three inches apart and arms form a circle at chest level. Shift your weight to your left leg and lift right heel.

SIX: Slide right foot behind left foot about twelve inches behind it, keeping right heel up. Lift your left arm above your head, and move right arm out to right side. Bend both knees; hold pose looking up at left arm. Tilt entire upper torso to the left.

SEVEN: Repeat step to each side.

To count with rhumba rhythm:

ONE	PAUSE	PAUSE
Step	Hold————Hold	

ONE	PAUSE	TWO	PAUSE
Slide	Hold————Hold————Hold		

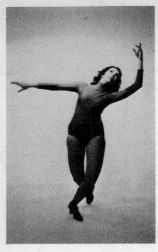

Step 35-6

Combinations: This step combines beautifully with many upper torso movements, and you should try your own combinations. Here are a few possibilities to get you started: 1. Combine simultaneously with Turkish arm pose (Step 22) and the head slide (Step 24).

2. Combine simultaneously with figure 8 of hands (Step 20) and spinal flex (Step 8). As you bring arms forward, contract; arch spine as you move arms back.

3. Combine with classic arms (Step 34).

4. *Challenge combination:* Combine simultaneously with snake arms (Step 33) and head slide (Step 24).

STEP 36—UNDULATING ARCH AND CONTRACTION

BODY TYPES: All, 4

Exercise: Mid-section, particularly for women after pregnancy

Music: Slow

NOTE: Review spinal flex (Step 8) before starting.

ONE: Assume starting position B. Stretch shoulders back; elevate rib-cage; keep legs straight. Lift one heel slightly and try to feel stretch from heel to shoulder.

TWO: Bend both knees forward, tilting pelvis up.

THREE: Bring shoulders forward. Rib-cage sinks inward; torso should be in contracted position. If you are doing the contraction properly, there should be a crease at the level of the navel.

FOUR: *Hold torso in contraction* as you push your knees back into straight position.

FIVE: Arch spine, raising shoulders back into standing arch position.

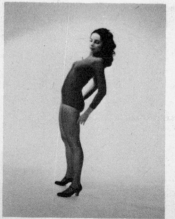

Step 36-1

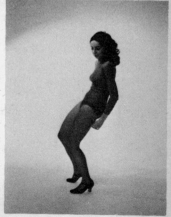

Step 36-3

SIX: Push shoulders further back; you should feel tension in the upper back. Lift rib-cage and start again from part 1 above.

Variations: 1. Proceed through parts 1 and 2 above, and *hold* position in part 3. Lift rib-cage while holding contraction, then release contraction as you straighten your body into a standing arch. This should result in a snake-like undulation of the torso.

NOTE: If you are receiving proper exercise value, you will feel vertical pull or tension through the abdomen.
2. For faster accent, do step as above (variation 1) but keep movements very small; abdomen should not move more than two inches.

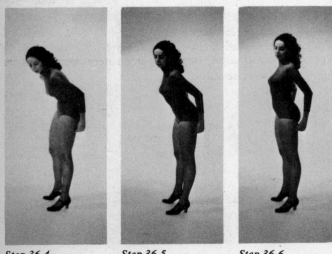

Step 36-4   *Step 36-5*   *Step 36-6*

To count with cifte telli rhythm: (X is fast accent)

ONE	PAUSE	TWO	PAUSE
One	slow Arch	and	contraction–

ONE	TWO	THREE	PAUSE
X	X	X	Hold

Combinations: 1. Combine with classic arms (Step 34).
2. Do step in kneeling position with Turkish arm pose (Step 22).
3. *Challenge combination:* Hold pelvic tilt (Step 11), and do undulating arch and contraction keeping body at tilt during entire step.
4. *Challenge combination:* Do *slow* forward arc of hip circle (Step 25), and as torso moves in arc, do four very small fast arches and contractions.

SPECIAL EXERCISE: This step is not usually done as part of a performance, but is included here because of its exceptional exercise value:

ONE: Assume starting position A. Keep knees bent throughout entire step.

TWO: Arch body, bringing upper torso forward so that your weight is on the forward bent leg.

THREE: Bring pelvis forward, contracting torso, and hold this position as entire body slides back and weight shifts to rear leg.

FOUR: Arch spine and slide entire body forward again.

STEP 37—HIP ROLL
BODY TYPES: All, 4
Exercise: Hips, mid-section
Music: Slow

ONE: Assume starting position B.

TWO: Slide hip out to left as in hip slide (Step 9); hold arms out at sides. Keep both heels on the floor. Keep both knees slightly bent during entire step. Do not buckle either knee!

THREE: Lift left hip, raising left foot so that toe just stays on floor. Keep right heel down!

FOUR: Tilt left shoulder down toward left hip. You will feel a contraction in the mid-section on the left side.

FIVE: Hold this torso position, keeping left heel up, as you push hips out to the right side.

SIX: Lower left heel, and hold exaggerated hip slide position to the right side. At this point both heels should be flat on the floor!

SEVEN: Lift right hip, raising right heel.

EIGHT: Tilt right shoulder down toward lifted right hip.

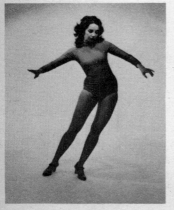

Step 37-2   *Step 37-3*

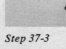

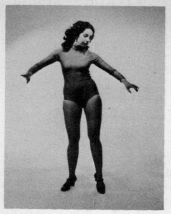

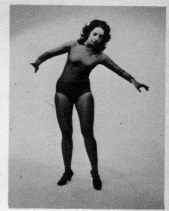

Step 37-4   *Step 37-5*

NINE: Hold position as you push hips into hip slide position to the left.

TEN: Lower right heel and hip slide to left side, both heels flat on the floor!

NOTE: Move hips *smoothly* in a horizontal figure 8; pause at each full hip slide with both feet firmly on the floor.

Variations: 1. For faster accents, do a smaller version of the step by sliding the hip only about two inches to the side.

2. *Counting with the rhumba rhythm.*

ONE   PAUSE   PAUSE
Slide to one side; lift hips slowly
and go half-way to other side

ONE PAUSE   TWO PAUSE
Small Slide Lift   Slide Lift

Combinations: 1. Combine with slow arm circle (Step 17).
2. Combine with figure 8 of hands (Step 20).
3. Combine with Turkish arm pose (Step 22).
4. *Challenge combination:* Combine simultaneously with Turkish arm pose (Step 22) and head circle (Step 24).

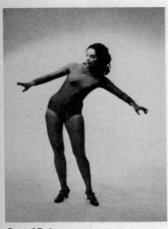

Step 37-6

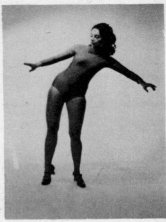

Step 37-7

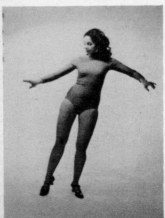

Step 37-8

STEP 38—HIP THRUST

BODY TYPES: All, 2, 4, 5
Exercise: Mid-section, hips
Music: Slow and bright

ONE: Assume starting position B with arms out at sides.

TWO: Place your weight on your left leg. Lift right heel off the floor; twist both knees to the left and bend them slightly.

THREE: *Thrust* right hip out to the right; slide shoulders to the left as in hip extension (Step 23). Knees should be only slightly flexed.

FOUR: Bend knees again, and repeat thrust. Also, repeat to the left.

NOTE: *Thrust* hip in this step, do not simply extend it. Use powerful thrusting motion as though using hip to push a heavy door shut.

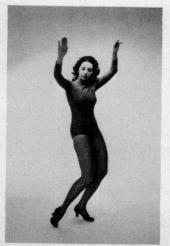
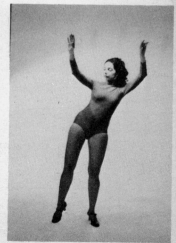

Step 38-2   Step 38-3

Counting with 4/4 rhythm:

ONE	TWO	THREE	FOUR
Thrust	Return	Thrust	Return

Combinations: 1. Combine with hip swivel (Step 10), and swivel hip into arcing position forward on each thrust.
2. Combine with slow arm circle (Step 17).
3. Combine with slow figure 8 of hands (Step 20).

Variation: Do smaller, *softer* thrusts to slower rhythms.

Counting with cifte telli rhythm:

ONE	PAUSE	TWO	PAUSE
Thrust	Return	Thrust	Return

ONE	TWO	THREE	PAUSE
Thrust	Thrust	Thrust	Return

Combinations: 1. Combine with very slow hip swivel (Step 10), adding numerous small hip thrusts as you arc hips forward and again as you arc hips back to starting position.
2. *Challenge combination:* Combine simultaneously with pelvic tilt (Step 11) and slow classic arms (Step 34). Thrust hip as you lower into the deep tilt and as you return.

Variation: **Step 38A** hip thrust pivot turn.

With your weight on your left foot, thrust your right hip; at the same time, turn on ball of left foot about one-sixth of a complete circle to the left (six thrusts to one complete revolution).

Combination: Combine with slight pelvic tilt (Step 11).

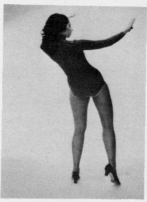

Step 38A-var.

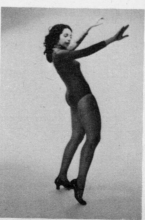

Step 38A-comb.

STEP 39—HIP THRUST WITH DEEP KNEE-BEND

BODY TYPES: 2, 4, 5
Exercise: Waist, hips, thighs, calves
Music: Any

ONE: Assume starting position B, with weight on right leg.

TWO: Bend knees to the right; at the same time, twist hips to the right.

THREE: Straighten legs as you thrust hips to the left. (Notice extreme shoulder slide to the right.)

NOTE: As in all steps of this kind, practice moving in opposite direction.

Variations: 1. Turn slightly on every thrust.
2. Practice with skirt (see illustrations).

Combination: Combine with pelvic tilt (Step 11).

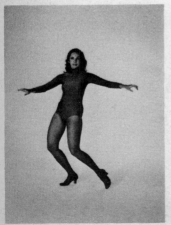
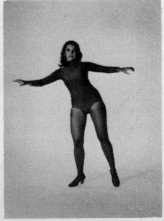

Step 39-2   *Step 39-3*

STEP 40—ANATOLIAN HIP MOVEMENT

BODY TYPES: 2, 4, 5
Exercise: Calves, thighs, waist
Music: Bright

ONE: Assume starting position B. Keep heels on floor throughout the entire step. This movement depends entirely on knee action.

TWO: Bend both knees as shown.

THREE: Straighten one knee slightly, pushing up hip on that side.

FOUR: Straighten other knee slightly, lifting that hip as you lower raised hip.

FIVE: Alternate lifting hips; vary tempo from slow to very fast. When done very quickly, this step makes hips look as though they were shimmying.

Variations: 1. ONE: Assume starting position B, both knees slightly bent.

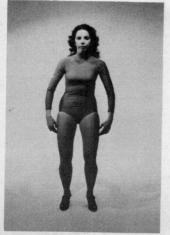

Step 40-2

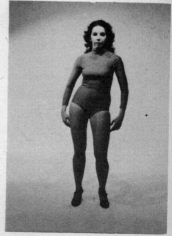

Step 40-3

TWO: Snap (stiffen rapidly) one knee straight raising hip sharply.

THREE: Snap other knee straight as you lower raised hip.

FOUR: Repeat smoothly parts 1, 2, and 3.

2. With both knees bent, place *all* your weight on one leg. With constant up-and-down movement of hips, turn in direction of leg bearing your weight.

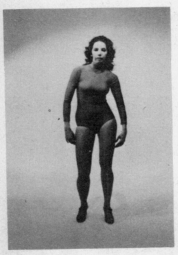

Step 40-4

Combinations: 1. Combine with very slow arm circle (Step 17) while moving hips *very* fast.

2. Combine with figure 8 of hands (Step 20).

3. *Challenge combination:* Using turn (variation 2 of this step) and very fast hip movement, combine with slow alternating figure 8 of hands with thorax twist (Step 21). Keep arms slow!

STEP 41—FLOOR DESCENT

BODY TYPES: All, 4
Exercise: Thighs, calves; balance and control
Music: Slow

NOTE: This step is quite difficult because of the control and balance it requires. When first practicing it, steady and support yourself with a chair, doorknob, or dance bar.

ONE: Assume starting position A.

TWO: Lift rear heel. Keep rib-cage high.

THREE: Slide rear foot back slowly as far as comfortable (see picture). As you bend both knees, remember to keep spine in slightly arched position.

FOUR: Slowly lower knee to floor.

FIVE: Return to standing position by placing all of your weight on leg that is forward; slowly straighten knees as you lift torso with spine in arched position.

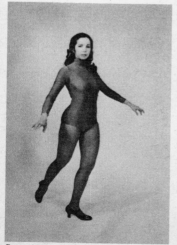

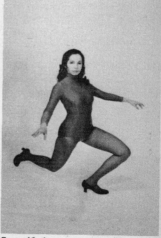

Step 41-3

Step 41-4

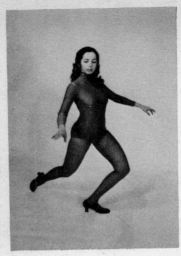

Step 41-5

Combinations: 1. Combine with slow arm circle (Step 17).
2. Combine with parallel arm circle (Step 18).
3. Combine with finger ripple (Step 31).
4. Combine with classic arms (Step 34).
5. Combine with snake arms (Step 33).
6. *Challenge combination:* Do step slowly and smoothly, adding Turkish arm pose (Step 22) with the head slide (Step 24).

STEP 42—FLOOR DESCENT WITH UNDULATING ARCH AND CONTRACTION

BODY TYPES: All
Exercise: Entire body; strenuous
Music: Slow

ONE: Assume position achieved at end of part 3 of Step 41.

TWO: Hold this position and exaggerate spinal arch.

THREE: Bring pelvis forward as you lower knees slightly; bring shoulders forward, and slowly contract at waist.

FOUR: Continue to lower knees, as you push torso back in contracted position.

FIVE: With knee about two inches from the floor, hold contraction as you lift rib-cage.

SIX: Release contraction, and arch spine as knee touches floor.

SEVEN: Return to standing position, with weight on forward leg, by rising part of the way on each arch; it should take a minimum of three arch-and-contraction movements to reach standing position.

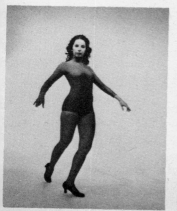
Step 42-2

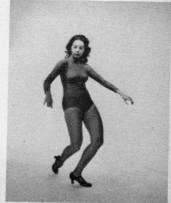
Step 42-3

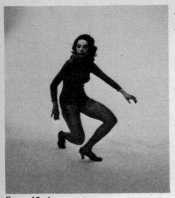
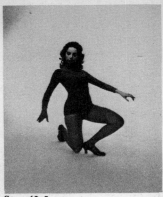

Step 42-4   *Step 42-5*

Variation: In descending and ascending, increase the number of arch-and-contraction movements, making them smaller.

NOTE: On steps such as this where the body movement is complex, it is best not to complicate it further with highly decorative or flossy arm patterns.

Combination: Combine with arm circle (Step 17).

STEP 43—BASIC KASHLIMAR
BODY TYPES: All
Exercise: Entire body; coordination
Music: Turkish 9/8 (see Appendix I—Music)
NOTE: Most steps, such as shoulder thrusts and hip thrusts, are easily adapted to this interesting Turkish rhythm. Because of its colorful effect, the 9/8 steps are traditionally saved for the end of a performance. In order to familiarize you with movements in a nine-count sequence, the Kashlimar walk is presented first:

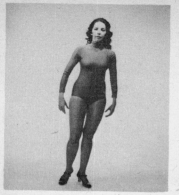
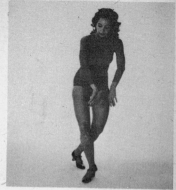

Step 43-2   *Step 43-3*

ONE: Assume starting position B, arms out at sides.
TWO: Walk forward, right foot first, with six-inch steps;
put a bounce in your steps:
BEATS:

1	2	3	4
ONE	PAUSE	TWO	PAUSE
Right	——	Left	——

5	6	7	8	9
THREE	PAUSE	ONE	TWO	THREE
Right	——	Left	Hold	Hold

BASIC KASHLIMAR

ONE: Assume starting position B, arms out at sides.
TWO: Place your weight on your left leg; lift right heel;
arch spine slightly to lift rib-cage.
THREE: Bring right foot forward about twelve inches,
shifting weight to right leg; at the same time, swing arms
forward as in figure 8 arm pattern (Step 20); contract
torso slightly.

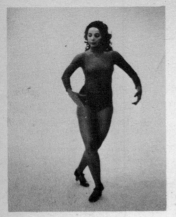 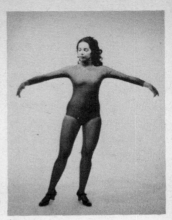

Step 43-4   *Step 43-5*

FOUR: Shift weight back to left leg arching body; slowly open arms out toward sides.

FIVE: Step about twelve inches to the right with right leg and shift weight to right leg, holding arms out at sides.

SIX: Slide left foot toward right foot.

SEVEN: When feet are about two inches apart, shift weight to left leg leaving right foot free to start entire step again.

To count 9/8 with above step:

BEATS:

1	2	3	4	5	6
ONE	AND	TWO	AND	THREE	AND
Step	Forward	Step	Back	Step to	Side

7	8	9
ONE	TWO	THREE
Feet together	Hold	Hold

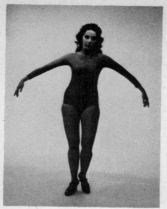

Step 43-6

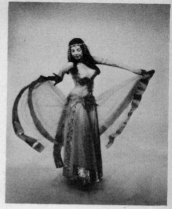

Step 43 var.-4

Variations: 1. In part 2 above, do a slight hop or skip on left foot before bringing right foot forward.

2. To travel forward, at part 6 above, slide left foot forward twelve inches in front of right foot; then continue as above.

3. To use as a turn, at part 3 above, bring right foot forward and six inches to the right each time part 3 is reached.

4. Do all steps as above holding skirt as illustrated.

5. Do all of above steps with a strong *bounce;* minimize movements so that feet barely move.

Practice other steps to 9/8 rhythm:

1. Step—point—step (Step 27):

ONE AND	TWO AND	THREE AND
Step	Point	Step

ONE	TWO	THREE
Point	Hold	Hold

2. Hip thrust (Step 38), first way.

ONE AND	TWO AND	THREE AND
Thrust	Lower hip	Thrust

ONE	TWO	THREE
Lower	Hold	Hold

2a. Second way:

ONE	AND	TWO	AND	THREE	AND
Thrust	Down	Thrust	Down	Thrust	Down

ONE	TWO	THREE
Thrust	Hold	Down

Do both variations of hip thrust with pivot turn (Step 38A) to 9/8 rhythm.

STEP 44—4/4 WALTZ
BODY TYPES: All
Exercise: Mid-section; increases flexibility of abdomen
Music: Medium or bright 4/4
NOTE: Though done to a 4/4 rhythm, the feet are accented three times for each four beats, thus the name *Waltz*. A real waltz is to 3/4 rhythm, which is seldom used for dancing.
ONE: Assume starting position B, with weight on left leg.
TWO: Step six inches forward on right leg; shift weight to right leg; lower right hip.
THREE: Shift weight to left leg, raising right hip.
FOUR: Step forward again on right leg, lowering right hip and lifting left heel.

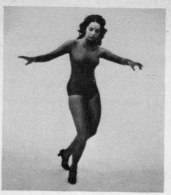

Step 44-2

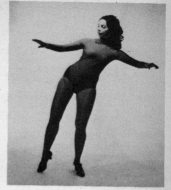

Step 44-5

FIVE: On ball of left foot, slide left foot in front of right foot; at the same time lower left hip.

SIX: Shift weight to right leg; lift left hip.

SEVEN: Bring weight forward to left foot; lower left hip, and lift right heel.

EIGHT: Slide right leg forward on ball of foot, and bring right hip down.

NOTE: On each full step there are three up-and-down shifts of the hip; each time you slide a foot forward, arc the hip on that side to a down position.

To count the waltz to 4/4 rhythm:

ACCENT
ONE
Step forward

ACCENT
TWO
Shift weight back

ACCENT
THREE
Shift weight forward

FOUR
Slide other foot forward

Variations: 1. Do step to the rear (backward). In order to get a smooth transition from forward movements, count as follows:

ONE	TWO
Step forward	Shift weight back

THREE	FOUR
Shift weight forward	Hold

Continue:

ONE	TWO
Shift weight back	Shift weight forward

THREE	FOUR
Shift weight back	Slide front foot back

2. As you slide right foot forward, arc it twelve inches out to the right; as you slide left foot forward, arc it twelve inches out to the left; each foot will complete one-half of a circle.

3. Repeat above, moving to the rear.

NOTE: Adding the arc to the foot slide is especially effective when wearing a long dance skirt, as it causes the skirt to swirl.

Combination: 1. Combine with slow arm circle (Step 17).
2. Combine with figure 8 of hands (Step 20).

STEP 45—FLOOR BACK-BEND

BODY TYPES: All, 4
Exercise: Thighs, back, abdomen; very strenuous!
Music: Slow

ONE: Refer to descent to floor (Step 41), and assume kneeling position with knees approximately ten inches apart.

TWO: Tilt torso back three to four inches with slight contraction at waist.

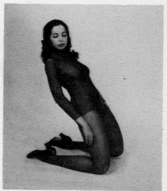

Step 45-2

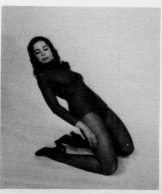

Step 45-3

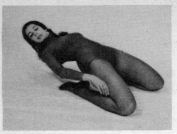

Step 45-4

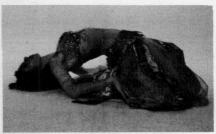

Step 45-5

NOTE: When first practicing this step, *stop* at part 2 above until your body becomes accustomed to the movement and has necessary flexibility. *Do not advance too rapidly!*

THREE: Continue lowering torso; as you do so you will feel great tension in thighs and back.

FOUR: Rest head on floor.

FIVE: Lift rib-cage, arching the spine.

SIX: Hold slightly arched spine position with pelvis leading. (Do not lead with shoulders!) Bring torso back to kneeling position.

NOTE: This step is a must for the traditional performance.

Variations: (See advanced section.)

Combinations: 1. Combine with classic arms (Step 34).

2. Combine with finger ripple (Step 31).

3. Combine with snake arms (Step 33).

4. Combine with shoulder thrust (Step 5).

5. Combine with kneeling parallel arm circle (Step 19). On upward part of arm circle, lower torso into complete back-bend.

6. Combine with hip thrusts (Step 38) to and from floor.

7. Combine with hip swivel (Step 10).

8. *Challenge combination:* Combine with undulating arch and contraction (Step 36).

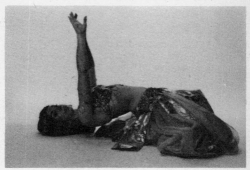

Step 45-comb.2

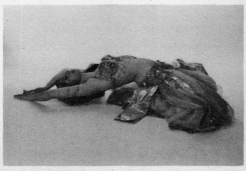

Step 45-comb.8

STEP 46—STEP—POINT—TURN

BODY TYPES: All
Exercise: Entire body; mild
Music: Medium, bright 4/4

ONE: Assume starting position B.

TWO: Place weight on left leg; lift heel of right foot. Step down on right foot. Spin on ball of right foot until you face fully to the rear. Barely brush floor with left foot as you spin. Do not raise foot too high or you will be thrown off balance!

THREE: At end of spin, carry left foot to left side, and point toe lightly against floor.

FOUR: Cross left foot in front of right foot; step down on left foot and spin, continuing to turn body to right until you face as in part 1 above. Keep your weight on left foot and point with right foot.

Variation: Complete entire circular spin on part 2 above, with arms at chest level and out at sides.

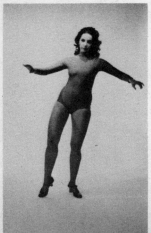

Step 46-2

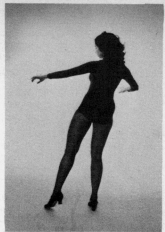

Step 46-3

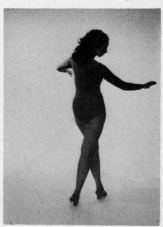

Step 46-4

Combination: Vary with step—point—step (Step 27), four step—point—step movements for each turn. Do not slow down turn! Keep in time with step—point—step, even at fast tempo!

Notes on Intermediate Routines

Even though the routines presented here are structured to provide you with well-balanced exercise as well as dance performances, you should remember: *(1)* that the dance is an expression of *you,* and that it is your creativity and imagination which make it come alive; and *(2)* that exercise needs are highly personal, and selection of steps depends to a great extent on your specific requirements.

Now that you have a greater number of steps to choose from and can put them together in more elaborate performances, here are some suggestions which will help you develop a more professional approach:

Transitions and Merges

A *transition* is the shifting from one major step to another, or from one type of activity or mood to another. A *merge* is a direct blend of one step into another. Transitions and merges are the glue of the dance and represent the art of coordination of all the elements of the dance. Though they can't be categorized as exercises in themselves, the control and effort necessary to make the dance flow smoothly constitute a major part of the overall exercise program.

No matter how well you are able to do a series of steps, lack of smooth transitions will give your performance a jerky, disconnected appearance, and you will seem to be a *catalogue* of unrelated steps. To avoid this, observe the general rule: Don't go from one step to another unless the movements are related; *i.e.,* that there is a point of action common to both. The only exception to this rule is the step which constitutes a period, or natural cutoff point, such as a sudden drop to the floor, from which you go on to a new sequence. For example, an undulating arch and contraction and a slow step—point—step are not compatible because there is no point where the two have a common position (pose) or movement. Therefore, it would be necessary to insert a step which complements both to eliminate the awkward choppy effect. The arch and contraction walk would be a good transitional step here, but it is an advanced step. Since there are many excellent transitional steps which you have not yet learned, you can substitute the method we call *overlapping*. This is a continuation of part of one step into the beginning of another, such as the footwork of the first step and the arm movements of the second. This technique is similar to the dissolve used in motion pictures, where two scenes are overlapped and the first faded out while the second is faded in.

Spotting

When you are executing turns, your head should not be rigid and *inch* its way around, nor should it just bobble on your shoulders. The most commonly used method of turning the head is called *spotting*. Hold your head still; fix your eyes on a point in the room (usually straight ahead); turn your body one-quarter turn; as your body continues to turn, rapidly turn your head so that when your body is three-quarters of the way around, your head is back at starting position; hold your head in starting position until your body completes the turn and faces forward again. This method not only adds grace to the turn, but because you are not aware of objects moving by, it also helps to prevent dizziness!

Buildups

Buildups are the crescendos of the dance. Starting with a basically simple step, such as a pose, more and more steps are added to it (and to each other) until the entire sequence ends in great excitement. Buildups are highlights of any performance and are crowd-pleasers because of the exceptional difficulty and skill they display. They usually consist of challenge steps and when properly done can be complete (and strenuous) exercise sessions in themselves. Though we will not go into detail here, think about the concept, and try to create some buildups as you practice the advanced steps. One buildup is given as part of the professional routine at the end of the advanced section.

Repetition

One of the basic problems facing every beginning dancer is: *how many times to repeat the same step.* Beside the stamina of the dancer, there are two limits as to the length of time a step can be done: *(1)* If not continued long enough, there isn't sufficient time for the audience to see and appreciate it; *(2)* but if done too long, it becomes monotonous. Most beginners are so fearful of boring an audience that they cut each step short and throw everything they know into the first few minutes of their dance, and then panic when they realize they have nothing left to offer!

Actually, the real test of a step is audience acceptance; as long as they continue to enjoy it you are safe . . . up to the point where you leave them wanting more by going on to something else. But it takes a great deal of experience to know exactly how well you're doing. Until you gain that experience, try the following: Prolong interest in a step by altering it slightly with variations, adding combinations, and spicing it with accents.

Pacing

As mentioned above, you can ruin a performance as well as an exercise session by exceeding the limit of your stamina. By practicing a strenuous step too long, you will find that you are too exhausted to continue to others which have benefits you need. Also, never overdo a difficult step during a performance just because you are getting applause; you will find yourself too tired and shaky to finish! Always intersperse steps which use different parts of the body from those you have been using, and which also allow you to catch your breath.

INTERMEDIATE ROUTINE 1 (SLOW)

ONE: Assume starting position A.

TWO: Combine snake arms (Step 33) with shoulder slide (Step 1) and a slow knee-bend; repeat four times.

THREE: Do classic arms (Step 34) four times.

FOUR: Continue classic arms and do slow floor descent (Step 41) to kneeling position.

FIVE: Combine floor back-bend (Step 45) with parallel arm circle (Step 18).

SIX: Slowly rise to standing position with parallel arm circle.

SEVEN: Combine Turkish arm pose (Step 22) with head slide (Step 24); repeat four times.

EIGHT: Continue head slide as you do Hindoo arm step (Step 35) four times.

NINE: Do hip circle (Step 25) once in each direction.

TEN: Do undulating arch and contraction (Step 36) twice.

ELEVEN: Do hip roll (Step 37) four times.

TWELVE: End with Turkish arm pose (Step 22).

INTERMEDIATE ROUTINE 2 (FAST)

ONE: Start with step—point—step (variation 2, Step 27), combined with figure 8 of hands (Step 20); do enough times to travel once around the room, returning to center of floor.

TWO: Do step—point—turn (Step 46) once in each direction.

THREE: Merge smoothly into 4/4 waltz (Step 44), forward eight steps, backward eight steps.

FOUR: Go directly to Anatolian hip movement (Step 40); repeat eight times in place; then with turn variation, once in each direction.

FIVE: Do deep knee-bend and hip thrust (Step 39) four times.

SIX: Do hip thrust with turn variation (Step 38), one complete circle in each direction.

SEVEN: Repeat part 6 above with turn variation; combine with pelvic tilt (Step 11).

EIGHT: Do pivot bounce (Step 32) with turn variation; end in Turkish arm pose (Step 22).

ADVANCED STEPS

Introduction to Advanced Steps

Congratulations! You have made it to the advanced level. By this time you are doing basic routines which are good enough to entertain an audience, and you notice a definite change for the better in your body and the way you feel. Yet it's at this point that Serena's sudents at the studio begin to ask very pertinent questions about the dance and what it may, or may not, have done for them. They have been so busy learning the steps and concentrating on their practice sessions that they haven't really had the time to stop and think about what all the hours they have spent with the dance will eventually lead to, and they wonder, "Where have I been . . . where am I now . . . and where do I go from here?"

Self-evaluation is always very difficult. It's not easy to be completely honest with yourself, and *nobody* can tell you exactly how to go about seeing yourself as you *really* are. In the past few weeks, you have seen a great deal of yourself and whether or not you are happy with what you have seen, you will probably agree that you have made some discoveries. One of the ways the dance helps you to learn about yourself is to present you with problems, and then to force you to examine yourself as you solve them.

Of course, evaluation means *comparison*. The student

is constantly comparing herself with the self that she was, the self she would like to be, and the self she sees reflected in the progress of others. How she makes her comparisons depends to a great extent on her personality and character. Those who are afraid of failure will manufacture success, and convince themselves that they are better than they are. Those who are afraid of the competition inherent in success will imagine failure. The rest of us are somewhere in between with our fears and fancies. That's why it's usually a good idea to enlist the opinion of a disinterested third party to add meaning to our understanding of ourselves.

WHERE HAVE YOU BEEN?

The question, Where have I been? really means: How well have I been doing? There is only one way to measure progress in the dance, and at the risk of sounding scientific in a discussion of art, we can express it as a ratio: Compare the rate at which you progress with the rate at which you are capable of progressing. In other words, it's a matter of efficiency. If you have been using all your capabilities and not getting anywhere, then you are simply slow. This doesn't mean that you'll never get there at all; it just means it will take you a little longer. It has been Serena's experience that many students who appear to be slow are really very painstaking and conscientious, and they often outdistance the initially faster students in the long run . . . much as in the old fable of the tortoise and the hare.

On the other hand, there are slow students who get very little from the dance because they operate at a very small percentage of their capabilities. They start with a know-it-all attitude, never take the dance seriously, attempt advanced steps before they are ready for them . . . and then wonder why they can't perform and why they are still huffing and puffing around in a size eighteen dress!

Stop now, and ask yourself: Do you feel better now than you did when you started dancing? Is your posture better? Can you honestly say you can do the steps in the preceding sections? Do you have confidence enough in your ability to perform them for others? Have you been enjoying yourself? Do you appreciate music more? If your answer to any of these questions is no, then something is wrong!

If you don't notice any physical benefits, then you have been making one or more of the following mistakes: *(1)* failing to put enough energy into the steps so that you feel tensions and stresses where you should; *(2)* cutting your practice sessions so short that you don't do the steps long enough to get any value from them; *(3)* allowing your inhibitions to prevent you from freely expressing yourself physically; *(4)* misunderstanding or misinterpreting the directions; *(5)* attempting steps before you are ready for them, making it impossible for you to do them correctly; *(6)* pushing yourself too hard; *(7)* distorting the steps by adding too much creativity too soon; or *(8)* rewarding yourself with banana cream pie and cheesecake.

If you see yourself in any of the above categories, by all means correct your mistakes *now* before you go on to the advanced section. If you have been skipping steps, or ignoring directions, or simply giving up on others, go back now and learn them. For one thing, you'll never get through the advanced section with an attitude of sloppiness, and for another, you'll never be able to do the steps since many of them depend on beginner and intermediate movements. Also, many of the advanced steps are well known by aficionados of the dance. You can thoroughly humiliate yourself by doing them incorrectly!

It's only natural to be discouraged from time to time.

At one time or another, every student feels that she has reached a dead end. It seems as though everything goes well and smoothly up to a point, and then nothing she does can improve her dancing. Many people give up at this point without realizing that the learning process goes in *plateaus*. There is no way to explain it, but people seem to learn rapidly at first, then suddenly taper off to nothing; then progress rapidly only to taper off again. It could be that the initial progress is so rapid that there isn't enough time for the material to be absorbed completely. Or it could be that the student burns up her enthusiasm and creativity and needs time for it to regenerate. At any rate, the plateau structure exists, and it is a test of the student's perseverance and maturity to overcome it. Success in the dance and physical development depend on overcoming obstacles, just as success in life depends on the same quality. If you take each problem as it arises, and solve it individually, you will develop a self-confidence that will enable you to tackle difficulties in other areas of life.

WHERE ARE YOU NOW?

Finding a disinterested critic is hard. Those who love you will tend to say things to make you feel good. People who dislike you may be cruel, in the guise of being frank, or they may flatter you in the hope that you will overstep your bounds and make a fool of yourself. So try to find a critic you can trust. It might be a girlfriend who is studying the dance with you; at least she would have some knowledge of the steps, and the two of you can correct mistakes in interpretation as you go along.

Sometimes, a husband or fiancé will make a good critic provided he is willing to be honest, patient, and impartial toward your selection of steps. Unfortunately, men have their favorite steps, and have a tendency to be impatient with those they decide are lacking in sensual content; and, of course, the value of a sexually aroused critic is debatable!

Do not depend on a teacher of another dance form to criticize you as a belly dancer! The steps in the belly dance are unique, and mixing them with another dance can be disastrous!

But don't set your sights too high. If you are reasonably sure you have a good understanding of the beginner and intermediate sections, and you can do the steps and routines gracefully, you are ready for the advanced section. There is no need to be absolutely *perfect* in the preceding steps in order to advance; it is the understanding of the fundamentals which counts. In fact, some students find that they enjoy the skill they have achieved with simpler steps so much that they dread going on to greater challenges; they relish being big fish in little ponds. This occurs occasionally in Serena's classes when students who are proficient as intermediates resist going to an advanced class where they fear that they will be almost like beginners again.

WHERE DO YOU GO FROM HERE?

Actually, the real enjoyment of the dance comes from the constant improvement of yourself and your skill, which almost answers the question, Where do I go from here? You can go as far as you want; the challenge never stops. There will never be a point in your life where you will not want to be, and feel your best. There will never come a time when you will not want to be active and sexually attractive and, hopefully, the day will never dawn when you will cease to accept challenge and abandon creativity.

By now, you probably know whether or not you intend to perform the dance for an audience (whether it's for a favorite few, or in a theater), and if so, it's time to start thinking about a costume. The costume section (Appendix II) will provide you with enough details to get you started. It's always wise to get the feel of a costume before you attempt performing in one, since many of the movements (especially shimmies and turns) are enhanced by them. It's also good to know what the problems can be, such as handling the bulk of a skirt, selection of shoes, and so on.

Proceed now, with the above in mind, to the advanced section. Remember that the notes and words of caution are based on the experiences of thousands of students, and are designed to help you. Good dancing!

STEP 47—SHOULDER SHIMMY

BODY TYPES: 3, 6
Exercise: Shoulders
Music: All rhythms and tempos
NOTE: Refer to shoulder thrust (Step 5) and note 2, Step 54.
ONE: Assume starting position B. Tilt torso back slightly (keeping body straight makes you appear to be falling forward); hold abdomen taut, arms down at sides.
TWO: Alternately move shoulders back and forth about one inch. Keep shoulders down, don't hunch!
THREE: Speed up shoulder movement until shoulders are moving very quickly: only about one-half inch forward and back. Do not move hips.

NOTE: Do not move arms and hands. Do not *shake!* Simple shaking requires no skill, and can be vulgar, especially in women with large bosoms.

Combinations: 1. Combine with pelvic tilt (Step 11) with arms held out at sides.

2. Combine with large circle of shoulders (Step 3).
3. Combine with kneeling sit-up (Step 13).

Challenge combinations (keep arms out at sides for all the following):
1. Combine with basic walk (Step 29).
2. Combine with step—point—step (Step 27).
3. Combine with floor back-bend (Step 45) (*very difficult*).

STEP 48—OASIS FLOOR LIFT
BODY TYPES: 2, 4, 5
Exercise: Hips, thighs, shoulders
Music: Slow
ONE: Kneeling as in part 1 kneeling sit-up (Step 13).
TWO: *Slowly* shift your weight to your right hip and assume position illustrated; right arm perpendicular to floor, about fourteen inches from right hip.
THREE: Shift weight to right arm; lift torso slightly. Right knee remains on floor. Continue raising body until torso is in straight line to the knees.
FOUR: Slowly raise left arm in large circular movement.

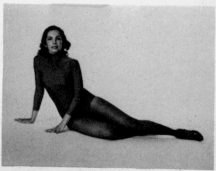

Step 48-2

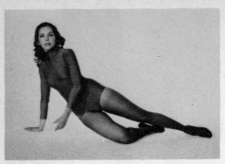

Step 48-3

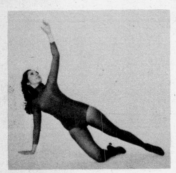

Step 48-5

FIVE: Stretch left arm high above your head; tilt head to look at extended hand.

SIX: Lower body as in part 2 above, and repeat, lifting torso again.

Variations: 1. Begin step with your weight on left hip.

2. *Oasis drag:* Start in position as in part 2 above, resting both palms on floor. Slide left palm to the right three inches; shift weight to left arm and slide forward with right hip grazing floor. Bring right palm to the right approximately six inches and shift weight to right arm. Slide

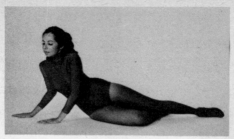

Step 48 var.-2

body to the right. Repeat until you have moved the desired distance. Practice also to the other side. (This step was popular in Hollywood "harem movies.")

Combination: Hold position as in part 5 above, and move left arm in large circle with finger ripple (Step 31).

Challenge combination: Hold position as in part 5 above, and do small undulating arch and contractions (Step 36).

STEP 49—BELLY ROLL
BODY TYPE: 4
Exercise: Abdomen!
Music: All rhythms and tempos
NOTE: This is a very popular step and is often misused. It is an authentic Middle Eastern step. There are two methods of performing it:

METHOD 1
ONE: Assume starting position A. Breathe evenly and naturally.
TWO: Elevate rib-cage; hold tummy in.
THREE: "Pod" out *lower* part of tummy.
FOUR: Keeping tummy podded, slowly pull rib-cage in.

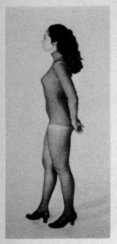 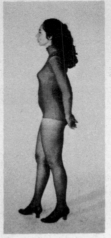 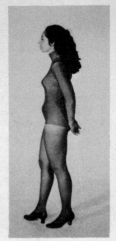

Step 49 method 1-2   *Step 49 method 1-3*   *Step 49 method 1-4*

FIVE: Slowly pull tummy in to slight contraction.

SIX: Holding tummy in, bring rib-cage forward.

SEVEN: Repeat to obtain smooth, rhythmic abdominal undulation. This step differs from the undulating arch and contraction in that pelvis and shoulders do not move!

METHOD 2

ONE: Assume starting position A.

TWO: Arc tummy forward and down by podding at the top and pulling in hard at the lower abdomen until you feel tension (about four to five inches below the navel).

THREE: Contract muscles in an ascending line as though a round bar were being rolled upward over tummy. As you do so, tummy should pod on both sides of the imaginary bar to create a travelling groove or indentation.

Variation: For both methods, alternate between very slow and very fast. Be careful not to be spasmodic or jerky.

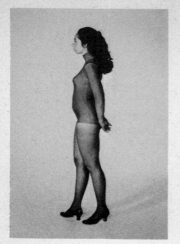

Step 49 method 2-2   *Step 49 method 2-3*

Combinations: 1. Combine with Turkish arm pose (Step 22).

2. Combine with slow knee-bends.

Challenge combinations: 1. Combine with floor descent (Step 41).

2. Combine with Turkish arm pose (Step 22) and slow step—point—step (Step 27). This combination requires great concentration and coordination.

STEP 50—DOUBLE HIP THRUST

BODY TYPES: 2, 4, 5
Exercise: Hips, legs, abdomen
Music: Slow and fast
NOTE: This step is widely used as basis for fast sequences.
ONE: Assume starting position B, feet at least twelve

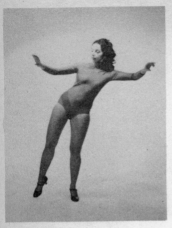

Step 50-2

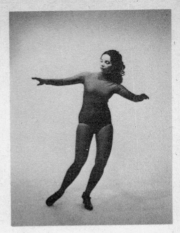

Step 50-3

inches apart. Place weight on right foot; lift left heel three inches off floor.

TWO: Lower left heel rapidly; *at the same time,* raise right heel and extend right hip as in hip extension (Step 23).

THREE: Hold position as in part 2 above. Bend both knees slightly to the left, and lower right hip.

FOUR: Raise right hip and *hold* hip extension.

FIVE: Lower right heel rapidly; at the same time, raise left heel and extend left hip as in hip extension.

SIX: Bend both knees slightly to the right, lowering left hip.

SEVEN: Raise left hip and *hold* extension.

To count with 4/4 rhythm:

ONE	TWO	THREE	FOUR
Lower right heel	Lower left hip	Raise left hip	Hold
Lift left hip			

ONE	TWO	THREE	FOUR
Lower left heel; Lift right hip	Lower right hip	Raise right hip	Hold

Variations: 1. For slower rhythms, soften and enlarge hip extensions.

2. For very bright (fast) rhythms the hip extensions should be very slight.

3. To travel, bring foot forward a few inches as you lower it.

4. To turn, move feet in circular pattern as you lower them.

Combinations: 1. Combine with slow figure 8 of hands (Step 20).

2. Combine with slow parallel arm circle (Step 18).

3. Combine with slow arm circle (Step 17).

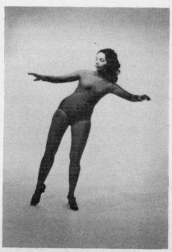

Step 50-4

4. Combine with hip swivel (Step 10). When extending hips on parts 2 and 5, arc hips forward as in hip swivel.
5. Combine with alternating figure 8 of hands with thorax twist (Step 21).

Challenge combination: Using footwork of step—point—turn (Step 46); arms out at sides; turn to left. Body faces to the rear on parts 2, 3, and 4. Continue turn to left on parts 5, 6, and 7 until you are facing forward again. Reverse turn, going to the right.

STEP 51—HOP WITH DOUBLE FLEX
BODY TYPES: All
Exercise: Mid-section, flexibility
Music: Slow, medium
ONE: Assume starting position B, weight on right foot; left heel three inches off floor; arms out at sides for the entire step.

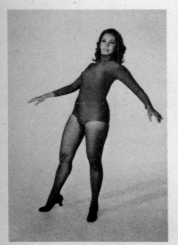

Step 51-2

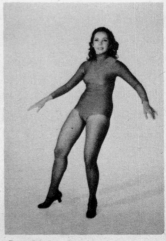

Step 51-3

TWO: Lower left foot quickly; at the same time, raise right heel, arch spine, and turn entire torso to the right. Hold this foot position for parts 3, 4, and 5.

THREE: Contract torso.

FOUR: Arch spine.

FIVE: Contract torso.

SIX: Lower right foot quickly; raise left heel and arch spine; turn torso slightly to the left.

SEVEN: Contract torso.

EIGHT: Arch torso.

NINE: Contract torso.

Variations: 1. In part 2 above, contract torso instead of arching; in part 3, arch spine; in part 4, contract torso; in part 5, arch spine.

2. To travel forward, move feet forward as they are lowered.

Combination: Combine with Turkish arm pose (Step 22).

Challenge combination: Keep arms out at sides. Use footwork of step—point—turn (Step 46). On parts 2, 3, 4, and 5 above, turn to the right until you face to the rear. On parts 6, 7, 8, and 9 above, continue turning to the right until you are facing forward again.

STEP 52—ABDOMINAL BODY SWIVEL
BODY TYPE: 4
Exercise: Hips, abdomen
Music: Slow
NOTE: Refer to hip roll (Step 37).

ONE: Assume starting position B, arms out at sides; slide hip all the way to right side.

TWO: Lift right heel, raising right hip; slant right shoulder slightly toward right hip.

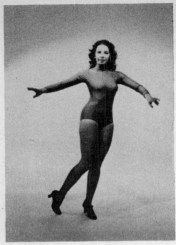

Step 52-3

THREE: Turn on ball of right foot twisting entire leg and hip so that raised heel points directly to the right. Keep shoulders facing forward!

FOUR: Slide hips all the way to the left; lower right foot; face hips forward.

FIVE: Repeat from part 1 above, starting on left side.

NOTE: This step should be done with a winding, snake-like movement.

Variation: For faster movement, slide hips only a few inches to the side; alternate between large slow movements to faster smaller ones.

Combinations: 1. Combine with Turkish arm pose (Step 22).

2. Combine with arm circle (Step 17).

3. Combine with slow knee bend.

STEP 53—HIP TWIST—HEEL AND TOE

BODY TYPE: 4
Exercise: Hips, abdomen
Music: Fast (bright)

ONE: Assume starting position B, weight on left leg, right heel lifted three inches, arms out at sides.

TWO: Twist on ball of right foot with right knee bent slightly, toes pointing directly toward left foot. Arc right hip to left. Keep shoulders facing forward.

THREE: Turn right foot to the right, straighten right knee, with right heel on floor, ankle bent to point toes upward. Turn torso slightly to the right.

FOUR: Bring right foot down quickly with a hop as you twist ball of left foot toward the right, left heel off the floor, left knee slightly bent.

FIVE: Turn left foot to the left with heel on floor and toes pointed upward. Straighten left knee, and face left with entire body.

SIX: Lower left foot, and proceed from part 2 above.

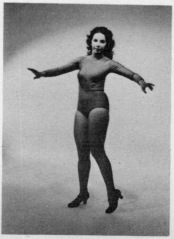

Step 53-4

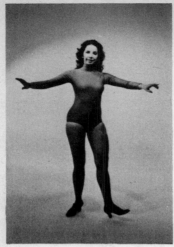

Step 53-5

To count with 4/4 rhythm:

ONE	TWO	THREE	FOUR
Right toe in	Hold	Right toe out	Hold

ONE	TWO	THREE	FOUR
Left toe in	Hold	Left toe out	Hold

Variation: To turn with this step, keep weight on one leg, and continuously twist the other foot in toe-heel movements while turning body to the right (or left).

Combination: Combine with slow figure 8 of hands (Step 20).

STEP 54—PELVIC FLUTTER
BODY TYPES: 2, 4, 5
Exercise: Thighs, abdomen
Music: Drum solo
NOTE: This step must be done with subtlety, often in sequence with other shimmies and vibrations. If the back-and-forth movement is too great, it becomes a vulgar bump.
ONE: Assume starting position A, both knees slightly bent, weight on rear leg, arms down at sides.
TWO: Tense muscles in rear leg; hold abdomen taut but relax derrière.
THREE: Bring pelvis forward about one-half inch.
FOUR: Push derrière back one-half inch.
FIVE: Move pelvis back and forth within one-inch distance.

NOTE: Remember that all shimmies depend on tension in one part of the body contrasted to relaxation in another. For example, in this step one leg and the abdomen are held taut (tense) while derrière and shoulders are relaxed.

Challenge combinations: 1. Combine with slow figure 8 of hands (Step 20).
2. Combine with continuous slow deep knee-bends.

STEP 55—KNEELING HIP EXTENSION
BODY TYPES: 2, 4
Exercise: Thighs, hips, waist
Music: Slow
ONE: Assume kneeling position (refer to kneeling sit-up, Step 13), with torso erect, arms out at sides.
TWO: *Slowly* lower torso so that you are sitting on your calves.

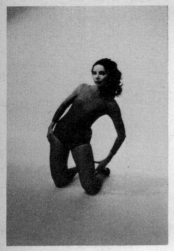

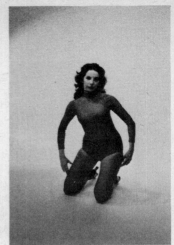

Step 55-3   *Step 55-5*

THREE: Slowly raise body to kneeling position; at the same time, arc hip as far as you can to one side. Extend shoulders straight out on side away from extended hip.
FOUR: Sit down slowly, arcing hip to rear.
FIVE: Raise body, arcing hips to other side.

Variation: For faster accent, hold hips out at one side; lower torso quickly as you arc hips to rear as if your body has dropped to sitting position. As you arc hips to other side, slow movement down.

Combination: Combine with slow parallel arm circle (Step 18). Hold arms overhead each time you extend hip to the side.

STEP 56—HIP SHIMMY

BODY TYPES: All

Exercise: Strenuous! Arms, shoulders, stamina

Music: Slow, fast

NOTE: Refer to hip swivel (Step 10), and practice it before starting this step.

ONE: Assume starting position B, arms out at sides, weight evenly on both legs.

TWO: Move into slight pelvic tilt (Step 11).

THREE: Tense muscles in upper-arms, shoulders, and shoulder-blade region.

FOUR: Arc each hip forward and back very quickly one inch. Keep arms still! Avoid making claws with hands!

NOTE: Remember to keep hips, thighs, and derrière *loose and relaxed*. Once started, the shimmy runs almost by itself and should appear effortless.

Variation: Hip movement should be *very* slight and subtle with slow music.

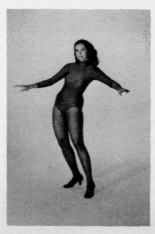

Step 56-2

Combinations: (Difficult!) 1. Combine with slow figure 8 of hands (Step 20).

2. Combine with slow arm circle (Step 17).

3. Combine with slow parallel arm circle (Step 18).

4. Combine with alternating figure 8 of hands with thorax twist (Step 21).

5. Combine with slow knee-bends maintaining pelvic tilt position on the bend.

6. Combine with short, rapid knee-bends to accent rhythmic counts (beats) as with 9/8.

7. Combine with basic walk (Step 29). Keep shimmy continuous and smooth as you shift weight from one leg to another.

8. Combine with heel bounce (Step 16).

NOTE: Many non-dancers ridicule the shimmy steps. They take the attitude that anyone can stand and shake her derrière. But the shimmy is not a shake. It takes great control, which the spasmodic shake does not. The good dancer makes the shimmy an art by adding fast hip movements to other difficult steps, keeping the shimmy continuous.

Challenge combinations: (*Very Difficult*) (Very Strenuous!)

1. Combine with slow hip circle (Step 25).

2. Combine with floor descent (Step 41).

3. Combine with floor back-bend (Step 45).

4. Combine with step—point—step (Step 27).

5. Combine with double hip thrust (Step 50) (very difficult and strenuous!).

STEP 57—VIBRATIONS

BODY TYPES: All

Exercise: Control, relaxation; a noted psychiatrist puts his patients in positions which cause them to vibrate thus releasing tensions

Music: Slow

NOTE: Vibrations are very effective in the dance and worthwhile as exercise, but they take time to perfect.

ONE: Assume starting position B, weight on one leg, arms down at sides.

TWO: Tense muscles in leg supporting your weight. Notice when you tense that knee-cap moves in and up.

THREE: Move knee of leg supporting weight back and forth rapidly only one-quarter inch, while continuing to hold muscles tense.

FOUR: Continue until vibration is achieved; shift to other leg and repeat.

Variations: 1. Do step with weight evenly distributed on *both* legs.

2. Tense muscles in derrière and shoulders, and vibrate entire body. The vibration still originates in knees as in part 3 above.

3. Experiment with isolated vibrations throughout body.

Combinations: 1. Combine with arm circle (Step 17).

2. Combine with parallel arm circle (Step 18).

3. Combine with figure 8 of hands (Step 20).

4. Combine with alternating figure 8 of hands with thorax twist (Step 21).

5. Combine with slow hip circle (Step 25); tense muscles in derrière.

6. Combine with slow knee-bends.

Challenge combinations (very difficult as you will be moving parts of the body in which muscles are already tense):
1. Combine with very slow step—point—step (Step 27).
2. Combine with slow descent to floor (Step 41).
3. Combine with floor back-bend (Step 45). Keep derrière tense.
4. Combine with slow hip roll (Step 37).
5. Combine with slow undulating arch and contraction (Step 36).

STEP 58—HIP SKIP
BODY TYPES: All
Exercise: Excellent overall exercise; stamina
Music: Medium-bright, fast
NOTE: This is a travelling step.
ONE: Assume starting position B, arms out at sides. Extend shoulders slightly to the left throughout entire step.
TWO: Step twelve inches to the right with right foot; at the same time slide hips to the left. These opposing movements are tricky! Practice them carefully.

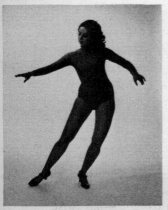
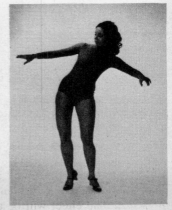

Step 58-2   *Step 58-3*

THREE: Slide left foot alongside right foot as you bend both knees slightly; at the same time, arc hips to the right.

FOUR: Straighten knees; at the same time, slide hips as far as possible to right.

FIVE: Repeat step as in part 2 above, travelling to the right. Always look in the direction in which you are travelling.

To count 4/4 rhythm (start at part 4 above):

ONE	TWO
Straighten knees, slide hips to right	Step right, slide hips to left

THREE	FOUR
Arc hips to right	Step right, slide hips to left

NOTE: This movement is from the *waist down!* Don't move shoulders!

Variations: 1. Do step travelling to left.

2. Bend knees *more* on fourth beat to accent rhythm and add lively bounce.

3. On *fast* rhythms do entire step on balls of feet.

4. Do smaller movements for faster rhythms; do greater arc of hips for slower rhythms.

Combinations: 1. Combine with slow arm circle (Step 17).

2. Combine with slow figure 8 of hands (Step 20).

Challenge combination (very difficult): Combine with hip swivel (Step 10); tense upper-arms and arc hips *forward.* The effect will be a travelling hip twist.

STEP 59—STEP—SLIDE

BODY TYPES: All
Exercise: Legs; with combinations, excellent general exercise for stamina
Music: All rhythms and tempos
NOTE: This is a very versatile travelling step, and combines with many other steps.
ONE: Assume starting position B, weight on left leg, arms out at sides.
TWO: Step to the right, about twelve inches, with right foot with foot pointed to the right. Straighten both legs *completely*. (This is one of the few times when both knees are perfectly straight.)
THREE: Slide ball of left foot to the right twelve inches so that foot is behind heel of right foot and perpendicular to it.
FOUR: Lower left heel and bend both knees.
FIVE: Repeat, starting with part 2 above, moving across floor to the right.

Variation: Reverse direction and travel to the left.

Combinations: 1. Combine with snake arms (Step 33).
2. Combine with Turkish arm pose (Step 22).
3. Combine with head slide (Step 24).
4. Combine with shoulder shimmy (Step 47).

Challenge combination: Combine simultaneously with hip shimmy (Step 56) and finger ripple (Step 31).

STEP 59A—PIVOT TURN

BODY TYPES: All
Exercise: Excellent general exercise; balance!
Music: All rhythms and tempos

NOTE: This footwork is used with many other steps.

ONE: Assume starting position A; right foot forward, arms out at sides, weight on right foot, left heel raised slightly.

TWO: Slide ball of left foot forward two inches.

THREE: Pivot to the right on ball of right foot one-sixth of complete circle.

FOUR: Repeat until you have turned full circle.

NOTE: Right foot serves as a pivot and stays in one place as it turns. Turn smoothly; don't bounce up and down!

Variations: 1. Pivot in opposite direction, starting on ball of left foot.

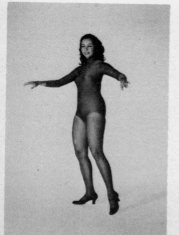

Step 59 A-1

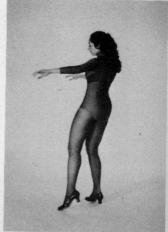

Step 59 A-2

2. Do step from starting position A with feet fifteen inches apart.

Combinations: 1. Combine with snake arms (Step 33).
2. Combine with alternating shoulder slants (Step 2).

Challenge combinations: 1. Combine with shoulder shimmy (Step 47).
2. Combine with hip shimmy (Step 56).

STEP 60—9/8 ROCK
BODY TYPES: All
Exercise: Legs; stamina
Music: 9/8
ONE: Refer to hip extension (Step 23); extend right hip, right heel off floor, shoulders extended to left.
TWO: Quickly reverse hip extension, stepping down on right foot; at the same time, lift left foot, extend left hip, shoulders to the right.

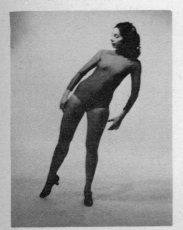
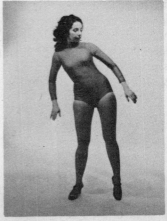

Step 60-1   *Step 60-2*

THREE: Step down quickly on left foot; at the same time, extend hips as far as you can to the right, and extend shoulders to the left.

FOUR: Repeat from part 2 above.

To count with 9/8 rhythm:

1	2	3
ONE	AND	TWO
Extend right hip	Hold	Extend left hip

4	5	6
AND	THREE	AND
Hold	Extend right hip	Hold

7	8	9
ONE	TWO	THREE
Extend left hip	Hold	Hold

Variations: 1. As you step down with right foot and extend left hip, lift left foot entirely off floor (only a few inches); do the same as you lift right foot.

2. As you step down with right foot, bring left foot forward six inches; at the same time, pull shoulders back; step down with left foot and move right foot to the rear six inches in *pointing* position; at the same time, pull shoulders forward. Repeat in rhythm.

STEP 61—TURKISH TRAVEL

BODY TYPES: All
Exercise: Legs! coordination and timing
Music: Medium, fast

ONE: Assume starting position B, weight on left foot, arms out at sides.

TWO: Move right foot eight inches in front of left foot. Turn slightly to the right; at the same time, bend both knees and twist them to the left. Shift weight to right foot; lift left foot slightly off floor.

THREE: Step back on left foot, and shift weight to left foot.

FOUR: Step to the right fifteen inches with right foot, and shift weight to right foot. Straighten knees.

FIVE: Slide ball of left foot alongside right foot. Shift weight to left foot.

SIX: Repeat from part 2 above.

NOTE: Don't move arms during this step!

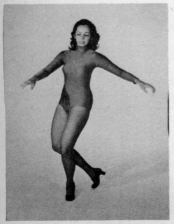
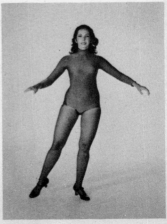

Step 61-2   *Step 61-4*

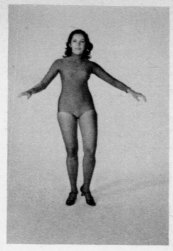

Step 61-5

Variations: 1. With fast music, do entire step on balls of feet.

2. Travel to left side. (Remember, you will go in direction of foot which takes the first step.)

3. To move quickly across a large room, take an extra long step at part 4 above.

4. At part 2 arc hips forward; at part 4 arc hips to the rear.

To count with 4/4 rhythm:

ONE	TWO	THREE	FOUR
Step forward	Step back	Step to side	Feet together

Combination: Combine with slow finger ripple (Step 31).

STEP 62—KNEELING TORSO SPIN

BODY TYPES: All

Exercise: Strenuous! excellent for stamina

Music: Slow

ONE: Assume kneeling position, knees two inches apart, weight on left knee.

TWO: Extend both arms to the left as illustrated.

THREE: Slide right knee ten inches to the right, shifting weight to right knee. At the same time, fling right arm out to right causing body to spin on right knee to the right. Tops of both feet *graze* the floor. Depending on the impetus of arms, you will travel a half circle, or full circle.

FOUR: Shift weight to left knee, arms out at sides.

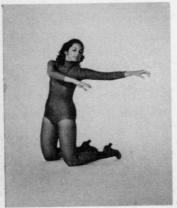

Step 62-2

Variation: Reverse above, and spin to the left.

Challenge combination (*very* strenuous!): At part 5 above, quickly lower torso into floor back-bend (Step 45). Raise torso and do multiple knee-spins and back-bends around room.

STEP 63—ARCHED STANDING BACK-BEND
BODY TYPES: 2, 4, 5
Exercise: Strenuous! thighs, back, abdomen
Music: Slow

CAUTION! Support yourself with a chair or other solid object when first practicing this step!

ONE: Assume starting position B, arms out at sides, feet at least 22 inches apart.

TWO: Arch spine as in spinal flex (Step 8).

THREE: Slowly bend both knees, and lower shoulders behind you; keep rib-cage high.

FOUR: Continue bending knees and lowering shoulders.

FIVE: Slowly straighten knees and bring torso to upright position while maintaining arch.

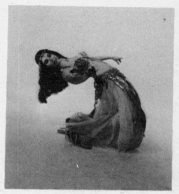

Step 63-3

Combinations: 1. Combine with classic arms (Step 34).
2. Combine with snake arms (Step 33).
3. Combine with shoulder shimmy (Step 47).

Challenge combinations: 1. (Very difficult.) Combine with slow, small arch and contraction (Step 36).
2. (Very difficult.) Combine with vibrations (Step 57).

STEP 64—CONTRACTED STANDING BACK-BEND
BODY TYPES: 2, 4, 5
Exercise: Strenuous! thighs! back! abdomen! great for developing balance
Music: Slow

CAUTION! Support yourself with a chair or other solid object when first practicing this step!

ONE: Assume starting position B, arms down at sides.

TWO: Contract at waist; slowly bend knees making sure that shoulders and knees are in a straight line.

THREE: Continue bending knees while lifting both heels slightly off floor.

FOUR: Continue lowering torso with heels lifted. At this point you should be balancing on the balls of your feet.

FIVE: Shift weight to toes, straighten legs slowly, arch spine, and maintaining arch raise torso to standing position. Then lower heels to floor. The rise should appear as though there were a rope just under the shoulder blades and pulling upward.

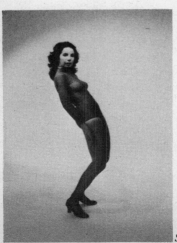

Step 64-2

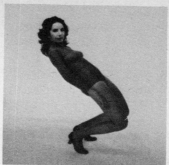

Step 64-4

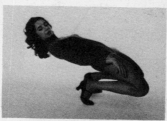

Step 64-Challenge Comb.

Combinations: (Because of the difficulty of the step itself, all combinations are difficult!)
1. Combine with shoulder slide (Step 1).
2. Combine simultaneously with snake arms (Step 33) and shoulder slide (Step 1).
3. Combine with classic arms (Step 34).
4. Combine with hip shimmy (Step 56).
5. Combine with vibrations (Step 57).

Challenge combination: (Extremely difficult! Practice over soft surface.) Continue *from* part 4 above; lower torso until knees touch the floor; at the same time, roll toes under so that top of foot rests on floor. Lower head to floor back-bend (Step 45).

STEP 65—DERVISH SPIN
BODY TYPES: All
Exercise: Excellent for developing balance
Music: Slow, fast
ONE: Assume starting position A, right foot forward, weight on left foot.
TWO: Extend arms to left as illustrated.
THREE: Step eight inches to the right with right foot; at the same time, *fling* right arm forcefully to the right, causing you to spin in a complete circle to the right on ball of right foot. Let left foot *brush* floor as you spin.
FOUR: End spin in position to start next step.

Variation: Spin to the left.

Combination (for slow music; balance is very tricky; be careful!): As you start spin, push derrière back. As you complete the turn, move hips into left hip slide position; then bring torso forward into hip circle (Step 25).

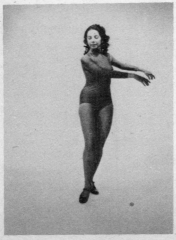

Step 65-2

Challenge combination (balance is very difficult!): Do *two* complete spin turns on one step, that is, go around twice with one push. Combine, then, with hip circle (Step 25) as in above combination.

STEP 66—FORWARD FIGURE 8 OF TORSO
BODY TYPES: All
Exercise: Excellent for mid-section; uses muscle not normally exercised
Music: Slow
NOTE: In order to do this step correctly, you must be thoroughly familiar with the undulating arch and contraction (Step 36) and hip roll (Step 37).
ONE: Assume starting position B, arms out at sides.
TWO: Slide hips to left in hip slide position.
THREE: Slowly arc pelvis forward; lift left heel and raise rib-cage.
FOUR: Slowly contract at waist; at the same time pull torso back slightly, with the left heel still raised.
FIVE: Hold contracted position, and slowly slide hips to right side.
SIX: As you reach hip slide position on right side, lower left heel and release contraction.
SEVEN: Arc pelvis forward, lifting right heel slightly; raise rib-cage.
EIGHT: Contract at waist; pull torso back slightly.
NINE: Hold contraction; slide hips to left.
TEN: As you reach hip slide position on left side, release contraction and lower right heel.

Variation: For a beautifully undulating step, alternate between smaller, faster movements and larger, much slower ones.

Combinations: 1. Combine with finger ripple (Step 31).
2. Combine with Turkish arm pose (Step 22).

Challenge combination: Combine with a subtle hip shimmy (Step 56).

STEP 67—9/8 CHA CHA
BODY TYPES: 2, 4, 5
Exercise: Coordination
Music: 9/8
NOTE: Refer to basic Kashlimar (Step 43).
ONE: Assume starting position B, arms out at sides, weight on left leg; arch spine slightly.
TWO: Bring right foot forward eight inches, shifting weight to right leg. Contract torso slightly.
THREE: Shift weight back to left leg; arch spine slightly.
FOUR: Move right foot alongside left, and put your weight on right foot; lift left foot slightly.
FIVE: Step down with left foot; lift right foot slightly.
SIX: Step down with right foot, shifting weight to right foot. Pause.
SEVEN: Bring left foot forward eight inches; shift weight to left foot; contract torso slightly.
EIGHT: Shift weight back to right leg; arch spine slightly.
NINE: Move left foot alongside right foot, and step down on left foot; lift right foot slightly.
TEN: Step down with right foot; lift left foot slightly.
ELEVEN: Step down with left foot; shift weight to left foot. Hold.

To count with 9/8 rhythm:

1	2
ONE	AND
Right foot forward	Hold

3	4
TWO	AND
Left foot back	Hold

5	6
THREE	AND
Right foot down	Left foot down

7	8	9
ONE	TWO	THREE
Right foot down	Hold	Hold

ONE	AND
Left foot forward	Hold

TWO	AND
Right foot back	Hold

THREE	AND
Left foot down	Right foot down

ONE	TWO	THREE
Left foot down	Hold	Hold

Variation: Each time you step down, *bounce* entire body.

Combination: Combine with large figure 8 of hands (Step 20) as used in basic Kashlimar (Step 43).

STEP 68—DEBKE STEP

BODY TYPES: All
Exercise: Coordination
Music: Medium tempo

NOTE: This step is adapted from a Greek folk dance step.

ONE: Assume starting position B, weight on right foot, left foot lifted slightly, arms out at sides.

TWO: Step down on left foot.

THREE: Slide ball of right foot forward six inches; tilt pelvis slightly.

FOUR: Move right foot alongside left foot and step down with right foot; at the same time, straighten torso.

FIVE: Slide ball of left foot forward six inches; tilt pelvis slightly.

SIX: Slide left foot to the left twelve inches, and step down with left foot as you straighten torso.

SEVEN: Slide right foot twelve inches to the left, resting it behind left foot.

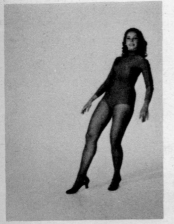

Step 68-3

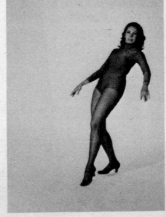

Step 68-5

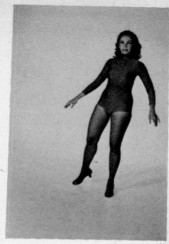

Step 68-8

EIGHT: Repeat from part 2 above, continuing to travel to the left.

Variations: 1. Repeat, travelling to the right.
2. Vary the size of the step from *very* small to large, with exaggerated pelvic tilt.
3. Add *bounce* to each step.

Combinations: 1. Combine with slow figure 8 of hands (Step 20).
2. Combine with shoulder shimmy (Step 47).

Challenge combination: Combine simultaneously with hip shimmy (Step 56) and finger ripple (Step 31).

STEP 69—HIP ROLL DIP
BODY TYPES: 2, 4, 5
Exercise: Back! thighs! legs! good for balance
Music: Slow
NOTE: Perfect hip roll (Step 37) before attempting this step.
ONE: Assume starting position B, arms down at sides.
TWO: Slide hips to left side, knees slightly bent.
THREE: Complete one slow hip roll (Step 37) to the right; complete one slow hip roll to the left.
FOUR: In left hip slide position, lift left heel; at the same time, raise left hip. Slowly *tilt* left shoulder toward left hip.
FIVE: As you begin to push hips out to right side, bend both knees deeply, twisting both knees slightly to the right. Push hips to right with both knees in deep bend. Lower left heel. Hold.
SIX: Lift right heel; at the same time lift right hip; tilt right shoulder toward right hip, with knees still deeply bent. You should feel tension in the waist.

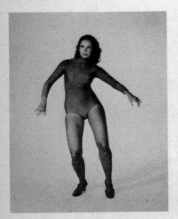
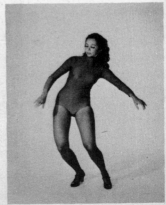

Step 69-4   Step 69-5

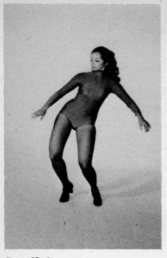

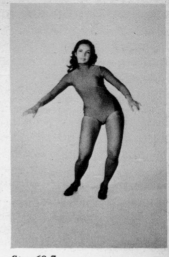

Step 69-6   *Step 69-7*

SEVEN: Push hips to left side; lower right heel.
EIGHT: Continue hip roll with knees bent.
NINE: Resume starting position by gradually straightening knees.

NOTE: This is a very popular step with professional dancers. It is often done faster by shortening the hip slide. When you practice it, keep movements smooth, never jerky. In shortening steps, many students develop a mechanical or wind-up doll appearance. Retain flexibility and grace.

STEP 70—UNDULATING ARCH AND CONTRACTION WALK (CAMEL WALK)

BODY TYPES: All

Exercise: Entire torso; coordination and balance!

Music: Slow

NOTE: This step is difficult! Practice undulating arch and contraction (Step 36) before starting this step. This movement is very popular and is characteristic of the dance. Since it is well known to admirers of the dance, be sure to perform it correctly!

ONE: Assume starting position B; with weight on left foot raise right heel slightly. Arch spine; stretch arms over head.

TWO: Push shoulders back; elevate rib-cage exaggerating arched position; at the same time, slide ball of right foot forward six inches.

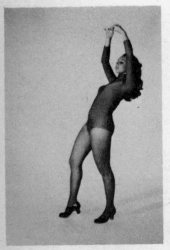

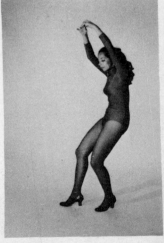

Step 70-2   *Step 70-3*

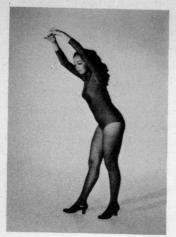

Step 70-4

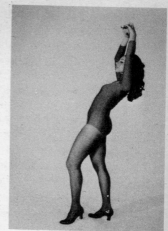

Step 70-5

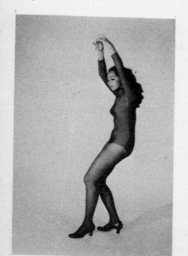

Step 70-6

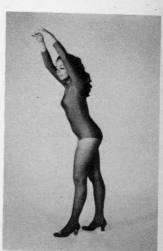

Step 70-7

THREE: Bend both knees, tilting pelvis up. Bring shoulders forward and pull rib-cage in. Torso should be in contracted position with knees bent.

FOUR: Hold torso in contracted position as you pull knees back until they are *straight*. (Do not bring right foot back when straightening knees! Leave right foot in place, and shift weight to it, as you lower right heel.)

FIVE: Arch spine and return to starting position B as you slide ball of left foot forward twelve inches.

SIX: Bend both knees; at the same time, tilt pelvis up and pull rib-cage in.

SEVEN: Pull torso back, holding contracted position; at the same time, straighten knees, shifting weight to left foot and lowering left heel.

EIGHT: Arch spine and return to starting position B as you slide ball of right foot forward twelve inches.

NINE: Continue from part 3 above.

Variations: 1. Do arches and contractions completely independently of the gliding walk. Integrate them as you desire, creating your own movements, but check in mirror to see that you do not lose original movements, as the results can be grotesque. Develop your creativity slowly and with a solid foundation of knowledge of basic steps.
2. Moving backward: *Method A*—Slide each foot back twelve inches *as* you contract torso.
Method B—Slide each foot back twelve inches *as* you arch torso.
3. For faster accents, use smaller arches and contractions with smaller faster steps.

Combinations: 1. (Extremely popular with professional dancers) Hold veil as in part 2 of veil arm circle (Step 28).
2. Combine with slow classic arms (Step 34).
3. Combine with slow snake arms (Step 33).

STEP 71—HIP CIRCLE WITH WALK

BODY TYPES: All
Exercise: Waist; balance, grace, coordination
Music: Slow

NOTE: Practice hip circle (Step 25) before attempting this step. As in hip circle, *do not* raise feet from floor—this is a *gliding* walk! Raising feet raises the hips, which, in this step, gives a very awkward appearance!

ONE: Assume starting position B, arms out at sides.

TWO: Slide hips to left, weight on left leg.

THREE: Arc hips forward, bending knees slightly.

FOUR: Slide hips to the right; as you do so, shift weight to right leg, sliding left foot straight forward six inches (not on ball of foot, but with entire foot grazing floor).

FIVE: Hold hip slide position to the right, knees slightly bent.

SIX: Arc hips to rear position as you straighten knees.

SEVEN: Continue arcing hips to left.

EIGHT: Extend hips to the left; at the same time, shift weight to left leg as you *slide* right foot forward six inches.

NINE: Hold hip slide to the left, knees slightly bent; continue step from part 2 above.

NOTE: For every half circle of the hips, the foot opposite the extending hip slides forward six inches.

Variations: 1. Move forward reversing direction of hip circle.

2. To move backward, slide foot back six inches instead of forward.

3. Add faster accent to either forward or rear arc of hips.

Combination: Combine with slow figure 8 of hands (Step 20).

Challenge combination: Combine with hip shimmy (Step 56).

STEP 72—HIP ROLL WITH WALK

BODY TYPES: All

Exercise: Waist; balance, grace, poise

Music: Slow

NOTE: Keep both knees very slightly bent throughout step. Do not let knees buckle! Practice hip roll (Step 37).

ONE: Assume starting position B, arms out at sides.

TWO: Slide hips to left.

THREE: Lift left heel, raising left hip.

FOUR: Slant left shoulder down slightly toward left hip.

FIVE: In this torso position, slide forward on ball of left foot; at the same time, slide hips to the right.

SIX: When hips are extended to the right, lower left foot so that both heels are flat on the floor.

SEVEN: Lift right heel, raising right hip.

EIGHT: Slant right shoulder down slightly toward right hip.

NINE: Slide hips to the left as you slide ball of right foot six inches forward.

TEN: Lower right heel to the floor as you hold hip slide to the left.

ELEVEN: Repeat from part 3 above.

NOTE: *Never* raise both heels at the same time!

Variations: 1. To go backward, slide feet back six inches instead of forward.

2. Add faster accents with smaller gliding steps.

Combinations: 1. Combine with torso movements of abdominal body swivel (Step 52).

2. Combine with veil poses as in veil arm circle (Step 28).

3. Combine with figure 8 of hands (Step 20).

4. Combine with snake arms (Step 33).
5. Combine with Turkish arm pose (Step 22).

Challenge combination (Strenuous for thighs!): Combine with hip roll dip (Step 69).

STEP 73—HUBBLE BUBBLE
BODY TYPES: 2, 4, 5
Exercise: Strenuous! legs, thighs, hips, waist
Music: Fast, medium 4/4, bright 9/8
NOTE: The term *hubble bubble* is another name for the popular *water-pipe,* or *hookah,* and signifies a bubbling, lively step, especially since the pipe was often filled with champagne. Practice the step—point—step (Step 27) and deep knee-bend with hip thrust (Step 39) before starting this step.
ONE: Assume starting position B, arms out at sides, right foot one inch off floor.
TWO: Bounce right foot to floor.
THREE: Lift left heel as you extend left hip to the left; at the same time, slide shoulders to the right.
FOUR: Bounce down on left foot; *at the same time,* bend both knees, twisting them slightly to the left as you raise right heel from floor.
FIVE: *Forcefully* thrust right hip to right as you slide shoulders slightly to the left.

To count with 4/4 rhythm (takes two measures of music to complete full step):

ONE	TWO	THREE	FOUR
Step down	Hold	Extend	Hold

ONE	TWO	THREE	FOUR
Quick knee-bend	Hold	Thrust	Hold

To count with 9/8 rhythm:

1	2	3	4	5
ONE	AND	TWO	AND	THREE
Step	Hold	Extend	Hold	Quick bend

6	7	8	9
AND	ONE	TWO	THREE
Hold	Thrust!	Hold	Hold

Variation: Start step with arms out at sides; at part 4 above, drop hands to hip level, palms facing rear. As you *forcefully* thrust hip, turn palms forward and bring arms back out to sides; palms will then face upward. As you repeat step, turn palms down to start.

Challenge combinations: 1. Use arm variation above and footwork of step—point—turn (Step 46). Turn right to face rear on parts 2 and 3 above; continue turn to right to face forward on parts 4 and 5 above.

2. On part 2 above, *spin* on right foot, turning very quickly in one complete circle to the right with weight remaining on right foot. Then proceed with part 4 above, facing forward.

STEP 74—DOUBLE HUBBLE BUBBLE

BODY TYPES: All
Exercise: Strenuous! legs, hips, thighs, waist
Music: Fast 4/4, 9/8
NOTE: Refer to deep knee-bend with hip thrust (Step 39).
ONE: Assume starting position B, arms out at sides, right heel raised three inches from floor.
TWO: Bounce down on right foot, as you deeply bend

both knees twisting them slightly to the right and lifting left heel. Hold.

THREE: *Forcefully* thrust hips to the left; at the same time, slide shoulders to the right. Hold.

FOUR: Bounce down on left foot, deeply bending both knees to the left and lifting right heel. Hold.

FIVE: *Forcefully* thrust hips to the right; at the same time, slide shoulders to the left. Hold.

To count with 9/8 rhythm:

1	2	3	4	5
ONE	AND	TWO	AND	THREE
Bend	Hold	Thrust!	Hold	Bend

6	7	8	9
AND	ONE	TWO	THREE
Hold	Thrust!	Hold	Hold

Variation: Turn to the right half circle on parts 2 and 3 combined; complete circle to the right on parts 4 and 5 combined.

Combination: Combine with slow figure 8 of hands (Step 20).

Challenge combination: Combine with hip shimmy (Step 56).

STEP 75—RUNNING STEP SHIMMY

BODY TYPES: 2, 4, 5

Exercise: Strenuous! legs! stamina

Music: Very fast 4/4 or 9/8

NOTE: Great as a finale step as it causes hips to shimmy even faster than regular shimmy.

ONE: Assume starting position B, knees slightly bent, heels off floor an inch and a half, arms out at sides, with mid-section relaxed. Keep heels off floor for entire step.

TWO: Bearing down *hard* on ball of right foot, move foot forward a half an inch almost as though stubbing it. As you do so, bend right knee slightly and straighten left knee slightly, causing left hip to move up.

THREE: Move left foot forward a half an inch in stubbing motion as above; as you do so bend left knee slightly, straighten right knee causing right hip to move up.

FOUR: Continue step from part 2 above, moving hips in short, sharp up-and-down movements.

NOTE: This step is *very* fast. On each measure of *fast* 4/4 rhythm, there are a minimum of eight stubs.

Variation: Do step in place, then move forward, then backward, then in circular pattern.

Combinations: 1. Combine with slow figure 8 of hands (Step 20).
2. Combine with parallel arm circle (Step 18).
3. Combine with slow arm circle (Step 17).

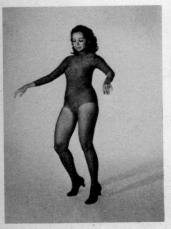
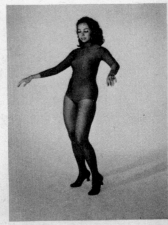

Step 75-2 *Step 75-3*

Challenge combinations: 1. Combine with shoulder shimmy (Step 47), arms at sides.

2. Combine with slow hip circle (Step 25). Make small circular pattern on floor with feet while moving hips in hip circle.

STEP 76—ARCH AND CONTRACTION PIVOT TURN

BODY TYPES: All

Exercise: Back!

Music: Slow

NOTE: Refer to undulating arch and contraction (Step 36).

ONE: Assume starting position B, weight on right leg, lift left heel two inches off floor, arm stretched above head for entire step, shoulders down.

TWO: Arch spine; slowly contract torso; at the same time, bend both knees and tilt pelvis upward.

THREE: Hold contracted position as you pull knees back into straightened position.

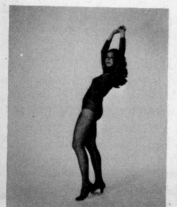

Step 76-2

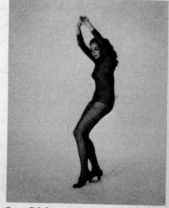

Step 76-3

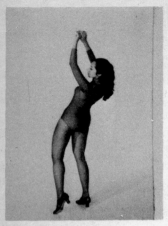

Step 76-4

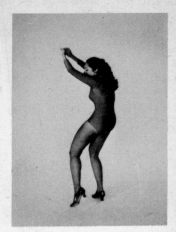

Step 76-6

FOUR: Straighten torso quickly into high arched position; at the same time, turn one-sixth of circle to the right on ball of right foot.

FIVE: Lower right heel, holding extreme arch.

SIX: Contract torso slowly; pull torso back while in contracted position until knees are straight.

SEVEN: Repeat, starting at part 4 above.

NOTE: It should take six undulating arch and contractions to complete one full turn.

Variations: 1. Turn in opposite direction, weight on left foot.

2. When you reach part 5 above, do two small, fast arch and contractions; then continue with contraction.

3. Each time you reach part 6 above, do *partial* contraction, and return to part 4 and proceed as written.

Combination: Combine with classic arms (Step 34).

Challenge combination: Each time you reach part 4 of step, do arched standing back-bend (Step 63); then continue to part 6 (skip part 5).

STEP 77—HIP CIRCLE WITH TURN
BODY TYPES: All
Exercise: Waist, hips, balance!
Music: Slow
NOTE: (Balance is very difficult!) Practice hip circle (Step 25) before starting this step.
ONE: Assume starting position B; slide hips to extreme left, arms out at sides, weight on left foot, knees slightly bent.
TWO: Arc hips forward, bending knees and stretching shoulders back.
THREE: Shift weight to right leg as you slide hips to the right; at the same time, arc left foot to the right four inches, grazing entire sole of foot against floor. (Don't lift foot!)
FOUR: Hold hip slide to the right.
FIVE: Arc hips to the rear, straightening knees.
SIX: Push hips out to the left, shifting weight to left leg; arc right foot to the left and back three inches.
SEVEN: Hold hip slide to the left.
EIGHT: Continue from part 2 above until you have travelled full circle and the turn is completed.

Variations: 1. Turn in opposite direction.
2. Add faster accents on either forward or rear arc of hips.

Combination: Combine with figure 8 of hands (Step 20).

Challenge combination: Combine with hip shimmy (Step 56).

STEP 78—BELLY FLUTTER
BODY TYPE: 4
Exercise: Abdomen!
Music: All rhythms and tempos
ONE: Assume starting position B, arms down at sides.
TWO: Inhale sharply, pushing tummy out.
THREE: Exhale sharply, pulling tummy in.
FOUR: Repeat parts 2 and 3 above, using much shorter breaths and much smaller, sharper movements of tummy: about one-quarter inch in and out.

NOTE: Try *not* to look as though *breathing* controls the step.
Challenge combinations: 1. Combine with slow hip swivel (Step 10).
2. Do floor back-bend (Step 45) until your head touches the floor, then do belly flutter (Step 78).

STEP 79—REVERSE ARCH AND CONTRACTION
BODY TYPE: 4
Exercise: Abdomen! back!
Music: Slow
NOTE: Very tricky! Refer to knee-bend with arched back (Step 14) and knee-bend holding contraction (Step 15).
ONE: Assume starting position B, arms stretched high over head, knees bent, and torso held in contracted position as in Step 15.
TWO: *Holding contraction,* straighten knees slightly.
THREE: Push pelvis forward.
FOUR: Stretch shoulders back; lift rib-cage exaggerating spinal arch.
FIVE: *Hold* arched spine as you bend knees; at the same time, lower torso, and push derrière back slightly.

SIX: At this point you should be in knee-bend with arched back position (Step 14).

SEVEN: Keep knees bent, and slowly contract torso.

EIGHT: Continue from part 2 above.

Variation: Use smaller, faster movements as well as larger, slower ones.

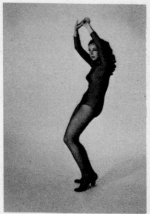

Step 79-1

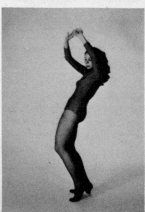

Step 79-3

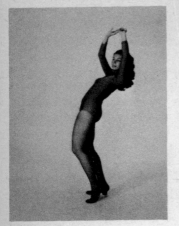

Step 79-4

Step 79-6

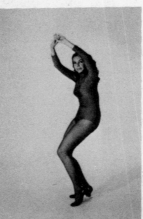

Step 79-7

Combination: Combine with Turkish arm pose (Step 22).

Challenge combination: Combine with floor descent (Step 41).

STEP 80—STEP—POINT—ARCH—EXTEND

BODY TYPES: All

Exercise: Very strenuous! back! legs! abdomen! hips!

Music: Fast 4/4 or 9/8

NOTE: Refer to hubble bubble (Step 73).

ONE: Assume starting position B, arms out at sides, right heel one inch off floor.

TWO: Lower right foot to floor.

THREE: Slide on ball of left foot four inches to the left, extending left hip to the left; at the same time, slide shoulders to the right.

FOUR: Quickly hop down on left foot, bending both knees and twisting them slightly to the left; as you do so lift right heel.

FIVE: Quickly arch up into arched standing back-bend position (Step 63); lean entire body to the right.

SIX: Straighten torso and proceed from part 2 above.

Variations: 1. Alternate by lifting left foot on part 1 above. 2. Skip parts 2 and 3; do parts 4 and 5. Straighten legs on part 6 and proceed directly to part 4, but hop down on *right* foot and reverse other movements in remainder

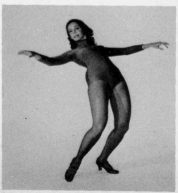

Step 80-5

of parts 4 and 5. Continue through part 6, and repeat all normally as written.

Challenge combination (Watch balance!): At part 2 above, lower right foot and *spin* to the right on ball of right foot in one complete turn. Then proceed at beginning of part 4 above.

STEP 81—ARABIC COFFEE MILL
BODY TYPES: All
Exercise: Abdomen!
Music: Slow, fast
NOTE: If not properly done, this movement can be *vulgar,* as it becomes a "grind." Keep legs gracefully bent to avoid the vulgar appearance.
ONE: Assume starting position B; extend hips to right, right heel lifted two inches off floor, weight on left foot for entire step.

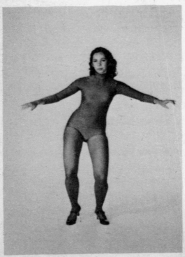

Step 81-2

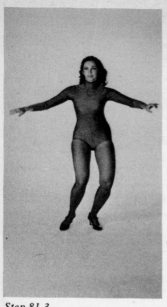

Step 81-3

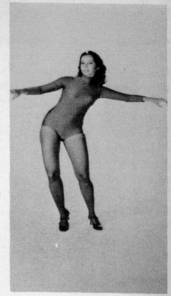

Step 81-4

TWO: Slowly bend knees; at the same time, arc hips further out as allowed by knee-bend. (Twisting knees slightly to the right will help.)

THREE: Keeping knees bent, twist knees slightly to the left and slide hips toward the left.

FOUR: Straighten knees; arc hips to right hip extension.

FIVE: Repeat from part 2 above.

Combination: Combine with pivot turn (Step 59A), turning on ball of left foot to the left.

Challenge combination: Combine simultaneously with hip vibrations (Step 57) and combination above.

STEP 82—HIP TWIST OPEN KNEE-BEND

BODY TYPES: All
Exercise: Strenuous! legs! hips! waist
Music: Fast 4/4, 9/8

ONE: Assume starting position A, right foot in front of left, weight on left foot, with arms out at sides; lift right heel two inches off floor. Feet remain in this position for entire step.

TWO: Bend both knees deeply, separating knees about eight inches. Keep right heel up!

THREE: Straighten knees; at the same time, twist right foot, turning ball of right foot to the left. Hips will automatically swivel to the left. Keep upper torso facing forward!

FOUR: Repeat from part 2 above.

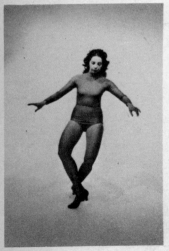

Step 82-2

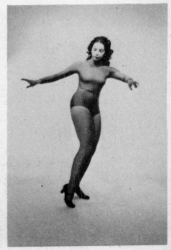

Step 82-3

To count with 9/8 rhythm (let X signify straighten—twist):

1	2	3	4	5
ONE	AND	TWO	AND	THREE
Bend	Hold	X	Hold	Bend

6	7	8	9
AND	ONE	TWO	THREE
Hold	X	Hold	Hold

Variations: 1. As you finish part 3 above, quickly reverse foot positions and go to part 2, but with left foot forward. Keep reversing foot positions on each bend.
2. As you bend your knees on part 2, turn to the left on ball of left foot. Repeat step until you have completed turning full circle.

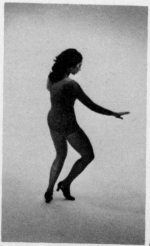

Step 82-var.2

STEP 83—BERBER KNEE WALK

BODY TYPES: All

Exercise: Very strenuous! legs! thighs!

Music: Slow, fast

CAUTION! Practice this over a soft surface! Be careful not to *bang* knees down on hard floor!

ONE: Kneeling position, arms out at sides, weight on left knee.

TWO: *Slowly* slide right foot forward on ball of foot, as you raise right knee. Pause when foot is alongside left knee.

THREE: (Difficult!) *Slowly* lower right knee forward to floor without moving right foot.

FOUR: As right knee touches floor, roll toes under so that top of foot rests on floor. Weight should now be on right knee.

FIVE: *Slowly* slide left foot forward on ball of foot as you raise left knee. Pause when foot is alongside right knee.

SIX: Slowly lower left knee forward to floor without moving left foot.

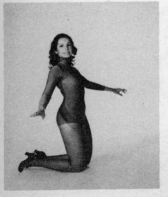
Step 83-1

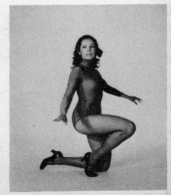
Step 83-2

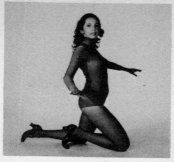

Step 83-3

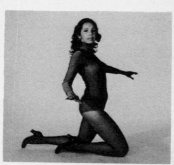

Step 83-4

SEVEN: As left knee touches floor, roll toes under so that top of foot rests on floor. Weight should now be on left knee.

EIGHT: Repeat from part 2 above.

NOTE: Practice until entire step is smooth. This will take time!

Combination: Combine with Turkish arm pose (Step 22).

Challenge sequence: Alternate with:
1. Knee slide (Step 30).
2. Kneeling torso spin (Step 62).

STEP 84—GYPSY HOP-TURN

BODY TYPES: All
Exercise: Strenuous! stamina!
Music: Fast 4/4, 9/8
NOTE: Study advanced routine notes: *turns, spotting.*
ONE: Assume starting position B, feet twelve inches apart, right foot two inches off floor, and arms out at sides.
TWO: Quickly arc right foot twelve inches to the right, keeping foot about two inches off floor.
THREE: Step down with right foot lifting left foot two inches off floor. *Hop* on right foot, as you do so turn body to the right half circle to face rear.
FOUR: Arc left foot twelve inches to the right, keeping left foot two inches off floor.
FIVE: Step down with left foot, lifting right foot two inches off floor.
SIX: *Hop* on left foot, as you do so turn body to the right half circle to face front.

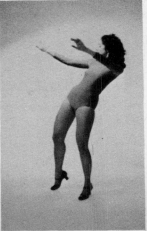

Step 84-2

Variation: 1. Tilt entire torso to the right on part 3; tilt to the left on part 5.
2. Take larger steps; hop higher, and when lifting foot, lift several inches instead of two inches. In doing so, you will achieve a *wild, bouncy* turn.

Combination: Combine with snake arms (Step 33).

Challenge combination: Combine with shoulder shimmy (Step 47).

STEP 85—FINALE DROP
BODY TYPES: 2, 4, 5
Exercise: Legs! coordination, balance
Music: All rhythms and tempos
CAUTION! Practice on soft surface! Protect your knees!
ONE: Assume starting position A; left foot forward, heel of right foot lifted two inches from floor; arms out at sides.
TWO: In one quick movement, drop swiftly to right knee; stretch arms high over head and arch spine.

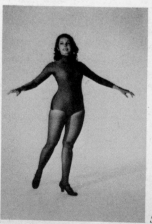

Step 85-1

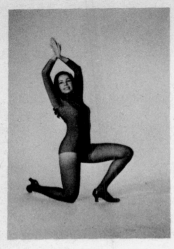

Step 85-2

Variation: 1. Alternate drop with right foot forward.
2. In part 2 above: while dropping to right knee, contract at waist and hold contracted position; kneel with forehead resting on raised knee, and combine with Turkish arm pose (Step 59).

Challenge sequence: Do three or four fast pivot turns (Step 59A) combined with snake arms (Step 33), and drop as above.

ADVANCED (PROFESSIONAL) ROUTINE
NOTES ON ADVANCED ROUTINE:

1. **The No-No List:** The following is a list of steps *not* to do:

A. *The Stripper Tripper:* The pelvic tilt position with a large forward and backward thrust of the derrière. It is named the stripper tripper because it is often used as a guide to determine whether or not a performance is obscene.

B. *The C. B. De Mille Special:* Berber reclining floor position (weight on one hip) while slowly elevating one leg high over head. This step is so named because it is a cliché of lavish harem movies.

C. *The Back-Splat:* Floor back-bend with knees facing the audience. It's an awful thing to do, and needs no explanation.

D. *The Titillator:* Fast shoulder-thrusts, with a forward tilt to the torso, usually within inches of spectator's nose. Vulgar. Invites trouble.

E. *Specialty of the House:* Floor back-bend with slow hip swivel and elevated pelvis. Tawdry step, highly reminiscent of shabby houses of ill repute.

F. *Narcissus:* Any pose, with hands stroking bosom, thighs, etc. No comment.

G. *The Nose-Wiper:* Gliding the back of hand under the nose, accompanied by great batting of eyelashes. Ridiculous. Another cliché of harem movies.

H. *The Flasher:* Any dancer who exposes herself. We didn't invent this one; *flashing* is a real word in the vernacular of show biz.

I. *The Vibrafool:* Reclining position with one or both legs rigidly outstretched and vibrating jerkily. It's a foolish thing to do.

J. *The Carpet-Sweeper:* A dancer who rolls around on the floor. Idiotic.

K. *The Indian War Stomp:* Great for Westerns where Indians are needed to whoop it up around the fire. Out of place in the sultan's palace . . . or anywhere else!

L. *The Shimmibore:* A dancer who does 45 minutes of shimmy variations. Ho hum!

M. *The Harem Globe-Trotter:* A dancer who walks, strolls, and trots about the floor . . . and does nothing else. No talent.

N. *The Hollywood Sphynx* (also known as the *Camel Driver*): One hand under the nose pointing forward, the other hand down at hip level pointing to the rear, with knees bent. Usually combined with a slow walk and a smouldering expression of the eyes. If you've ever smelled a camel, you'll know why the hand protects the nose, and the eyes are smouldering. This step has an aroma, too.

O. *The Fig-Plucker:* Any step accompanied by fast, jerky up-and-down reach of the arms. Hilarious on the dance floor, but great for hailing taxis.

2. *Reminders:*

A. Replace steps with others when they seem to fit your body type and personality better. Innovate!

B. Never perform a step for any audience until you are sure you can do it well.

C. Be very conscious of your posture; be proud and sure of yourself. Keep your shoulders down and rib-cage high.

D. Always reflect the purest principles of the dance; make certain that none of your movements are vulgar in any way.

E. Avoid clichés and artificiality.

F. Maintain contact with your audience by warmly expressing your personality. Don't make faces which betray the fact that you are having problems.

G. Put plenty of variety in your dance. Move around; don't do all your dancing in one place or direct it at one small group of people.

H. Use your veil!

ADVANCED (PROFESSIONAL) ROUTINE:

Music: Fast

1. Drape veil around torso before entering.

2. Enter fast with travelling variation of double hip thrust (Step 50) combined with figure 8 of hands (Step 20). Go around room once, to end in center.

3. Do hip thrust (Step 38) combined with arm circle (Step 17), twice to the right and twice to the left.

4. Do heel bounce variation of hip circle (Step 25) combined with figure 8 of hands (Step 20); two hip circles to the right; two to the left.

5. Do hip skip (Step 58) combined with slow arm circle (Step 17) once around the room.

6. Do step—point—step (Step 27), arms out at sides, forward eight steps, backward eight steps.

7. Do step—point—turn (Step 46), arms out at sides, once to left, once to right.

8. Do hubble bubble (Step 73) twice.

9. Do double hubble bubble (Step 74) four times.

10. Do fast pivot turn (Step 59A) combined with snake arms (Step 33) twice; then slow down to end in Turkish arm pose (Step 22).

Music: Slow, veil dance

11. Do classic arms (Step 34) four times.

12. Do alternating figure 8 of hands with thorax twist (Step 21) twice.

13. Do parallel arm circle (Step 18) once to each side.

14. Do hip circle (Step 25) combined with figure 8 of hands (Step 20) once in each direction.

15. Do hip circle with turn (Step 77) two complete turns while continuing figure 8 of hands from above.

16. Do hip roll (Step 37), arms out at sides, twice.

17. Alternate hip roll (Step 37) with hip roll dip (Step 69) while unfastening veil. Do not discard veil.

18. Do veil arm circle (Step 28) once in each direction.

19. Hold veil in front of you and do arch and contraction walk (Step 70) forward eight steps, and with veil held behind you, back eight steps. Still holding veil behind you, do reverse arch and contraction (Step 79) twice, and drop veil to floor.

20. Slowly stretch arms high over head and do hip roll with walk (Step 72) forward six steps, backward six steps.

21. Merge to abdominal body swivel (Step 52), arms out at sides, four times.

22. Do forward figure 8 of torso (Step 66), arms still out at sides.

Music: Slow, floor work

23. Do descent to floor with arch and contraction (Step 42) combined with classic arms (Step 34).

24. In kneeling position, do snake arms (Step 33) combined with shoulder slide (Step 1) twice.

25. Continue snake arms (as above) into floor back-bend (Step 35).

26. Slowly return to kneeling position, and do knee slides (Step 30) with parallel arm circle (Step 18) twice in each direction.

27. Do kneeling torso spin (Step 62) three times.

28. Do *very* slow floor back-bend (Step 45) combined with classic arms (Step 34).

29. Hold back-bend, head resting on floor, arms stretched back beyond head; combine with arch and contraction (Step 36) using faster accent variation.

30. Do belly flutter (Step 78) while in back-bend.

31. Slowly rise from floor to kneeling position, with spine in arched position.

32. Return to standing position with small arch and contraction (Step 36); stretch arms high over head.

33. Do finger ripple (Step 31) with arms still over head; combine with belly roll (Step 49) with alternating faster accents.

34. Go into slow step—point—step (Step 27) continuing finger ripple.

Music: Fast

35. Accelerate step—point—step to bouncy fast. Do four forward, four backward to fast rhythm.

36. Do Turkish travel (Step 61) combined with arm circle (Step 17) and move around edge of room once; return to center of floor.

37. Do deep knee-bend and hip thrust (Step 39) using turn variation once in each direction.

38. Merge into 4/4 waltz (Step 44) arms out at sides; forward eight steps, backward eight steps.

39. Do hip circle (Step 25) combined with heel bounce (Step 16).

Music: 9/8; if no 9/8 do steps to 4/4; review method

40. Hip circle combined with heel bounce (as above) to 9/8 rhythm.

41. Basic Kashlimar (Step 43) using skirt as illustrated, and hop variation. Travel around edge of room with this step, returning to center.

42. Do hubble bubble (Step 73) arms out at sides.

43. Do hip twist with open knee-bend (Step 82) six measures of music, as you turn.

44. Do hip thrust (Step 38) with hip swivel variation, four times.

45. Merge to Anatolian hips (Step 40), four measures of music.

NOTE: Steps 45, 46, 47, 48, and 49 below constitute a buildup.

46. Do hip shimmy (Step 56) arms out at sides, combined with small knee-bends to accent rhythm.

47. Continue hip shimmy, moving torso into pelvic tilt position (Step 11).

48. Continue hip shimmy, moving torso into contracted standing back-bend (Step 64).

49. Hold position, varying size of shimmy for four measures, accent rhythm with small knee-bends.

50. Continue shimmy, and raise torso to standing position.

51. Do basic Kashlimar (Step 43) combined with hip shimmy; use skirt; circle room, and return to center of floor.

52. Do running step shimmy (Step 75) holding skirt out at sides.

53. Continue running step shimmy combined with hip twist (Step 12) to accent rhythm.

54. Continue holding skirt out at sides, and do fast pivot turn (Step 59A) three times.

55. Do finale drop (Step 84) combined with Turkish arm pose (Step 22).

56. Exit gracefully to roars of applause!

APPENDIX I

MUSIC

1. *Glossary of Musical Terms:*

A. *Beat*—Unit of rhythm; as 4 beats to measure of 4/4 time:

One measure   One measure
One–two–three–four / One–two–three–four

B. *Bright:* Used to indicate the *way* in which a composition is to be played; cheerfully, animatedly lively.

C. *Chorus:* The refrain of a song, following the verse. Usually the better known portion of a song; often used by dancers to indicate the length of time a composition is to be played: "Play two choruses of Misirlou."

D. *Key:* The group of notes or tones comprising a *scale* or main tonality of a composition; based on and named after a note of the scale.

E. *Measure (bar):* The space between two vertical lines which contains the number of notes given in the time signature.

F. *Mode:* Scales in various arrangements of tones as in classical Greek and Medieval church music. Much Oriental music is written in modes, accounting in part for the distinctive sound.

G. *Rhythm:* A pattern of regularly recurring accents, or "beats." In contrast to periodicity, in which the recurrent tone has no emphasis, rhythm exists because of accents. Literally, rhythm is "measured motion" and as such forms the framework of dance.

H. *Segue:* By definition, to perform a part of a work in the manner of a preceding part. In common usage, to go from one song to another smoothly and without a pause.

I. *Syncopation:* Shifting of accents to normally unaccented positions.

J. *Tempo:* The *speed* at which a composition is played. A *rhythm* can be played at a variety of tempos.

K. *Time:* The number and kind of notes in each measure:

Examples: $4/4 = \dfrac{\text{four}}{\text{quarter notes}}$ $9/8 = \dfrac{\text{nine}}{\text{eighth notes}}$

This term is sometimes used to indicate rhythm, as in "Waltz Time," etc.

2. *Rhythms Used in the Dance:*

A. *4/4:* Approximately half of the dance, when done as a performance, will be to a fast 4/4 rhythm. The placement of the accents must be as follows:

ONE two THREE four / ONE two THREE four

You will notice that beats ONE and THREE receive an accent, or "punch," that the others do not. In accenting, be careful not to give extra time value to the first and third beats! This is often called "cut" time since the effect is similar to the rhythm 2/4: ONE two/ONE two. Most rock and roll and jazz will provide you with excellent 4/4 practice rhythms.

B. *Cifte Telli:* This is a 4/4 rhythm which requires two measures of music to complete. Even though it has four beats to the measure, the placement of the accents gives it a unique sound. Practice it while reciting the nonsense words written below:

1	2	3	4
BOOM	pa-pa	pa-pa	paaaaa
I	am a	little	bird I

1	2	3	4
BOOM	BOOM	BOOM	PAUSE
fly	over	you	

This is a slow rhythm; if you don't have a record of it, practice with a rhumba or slow ballad.

C. *Rhumba:* The slow rhumba as used in the dance is accented differently from the American version, however the number of beats is the same . . . four to the measure with two measures required to complete it. Practice as follows:

1	2	3	4	1	2	3	4
BOOM	Paa-	aaa	paaa	BOOM		paa-aaa	
I	am		a	Dan-		cer	

D. *Kashlimar:* There is no counterpart to the 9/8 Turkish rhythm in American music, so it won't be found on the radio where American music is featured. However, you can count it to yourself as follows:

1 2	3 4	5 6	7	8	9
ONE	TWO	THREE	ONE	two	three

Place your accents as above, or if you are counting all nine beats the accents would fall on beats 1—3—5—7. Sometimes the rhythm will be played so that you will not hear beats 8 and 9, but even though they are not *heard,* they are still *counted.*

E. *Taksim:* There is no counterpart in American music for this. It is highly interpretive, and flowing, *without* a time signature; that is, it has no definite number of beats in a given time. Usually performed as a solo. Makes an excellent accompaniment for slow, fluid movements and is a favorite for floor work.

F. *Other rhythms:* If you purchase a record of Middle Eastern music, you will probably find strange rhythms, such as 7/8, 5/4, 6/8, etc. on it. Do not attempt to dance to these until you know exactly what you are doing! They will confuse you, and make it impossible for you to learn the steps.

3. *Playing the Zills:*

Study the zill positions as shown in the diagrams. Then, attempt the various sounds described below:

Position 1—The zills are struck evenly face-to-face and released quickly. This will result in a "ringing" sound.

Position 2—The zills are struck as in 1, but held tightly together, or "damped" by pressing the index and ring fingers against the zills. This will result in a dull clacking sound.

Position 3—The zills are brought together in arcs, so that only the outer rims touch. The contact is extremely brief, so that a tinging sound is produced.

Position 4—Zills are damped, as in 2, except that thumb zill is also softened by holding it against base of index finger. This results in a light clicking sound.

Position 5—This is a trilling sound produced by *raking* the edges of one pair of zills over the edges of another.

In practicing the following rhythms, you *must* play the accents as they are given; however, use as much imagination as you can in varying the *sound* of the zills:

Fast 4/4:

	1	2	3	4
A.	PING	ta ta	PING	PING
	L	R R	L	R

	1	2	3	4
B.	PING	ta ta	ta ta	ta ta
	L	R R	L L	R R

	1	2	3	4
C.	Ta ta	ta ta	ta ta	ta ta
	L R	L R	L R	L R

Cifte Telli:

	1	2	3	4
A.	PING	ta ta	ta ta	PING
	L	R R	L L	R

	1	2	3	4
	RING	RING	RING	(Pause)
	R	L	R	

	1	2	3	4
B.	PING	ta ta	ta ta	ta ta/
	L	R R R	L L	R R

	1	2	3	4
	RING	RING	RING	ta ta
	L	R	L	R R

Rhumba:

	1	2 3	4 1 2	3 4
A.	PING	taaaaaa	taaa／RING	RING
	L	R	R L	R

	1	2	3	4 1 2	3 4
B.	PING	tata	taaaaaa	taaa／Ping	Ping
	L	RR	L	R L	R

Kashlimar:

	1 2	3 4	5 6	7	8	9
A.	PING	PING	PING	ta	ta	ta
	L	R	L	R	L	R

	1	2	3	4	5	6	7	8	9
B.	ta	ta	ta	ta	ta	ta	ta	ta	ta
	L	R	L	R	L	R	L	R	R

(Accents on 1,3,5,7)

NOTES:

A. The left–right hand movements need not be followed as written. They are only indicated as an aid in getting started. You can change them around as you like if you find it easier to play another way.

B. As you have noticed, a simple "ta" is equivalent to one-half of a PING. Therefore, you can play two "ta" sounds for each PING. For example: PING PING PING PING could be played ta ta ta ta ta ta ta ta; provided, of course, the amount of time required to play each is the same.

C. If you play the zills with a taksim, you can play what-ever you wish so long as it goes with your movements and

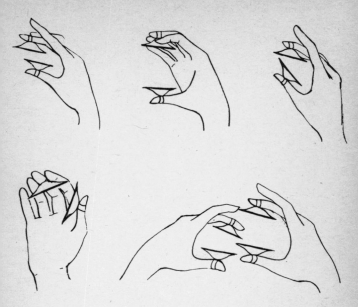

is not obtrusive. However, a gentle, continuous, clicking sound is best; you can accent it as you wish.

D. Do not overplay the zills! They are a musical instrument and should complement your dance and the music. They can be used to produce buildups, and the volume can be varied (shaded) for dramatic effects. Avoid the "doorbell" or random, incessant, clanging sound!

4. *Selecting Music:*

If you are to perform with records or tape, the music will always be just as you want it. However, if you are dancing to the music of live musicians, you will have to choose music that they can play with little or no rehearsal. For this reason it is best to give them a sheet of paper containing a list of songs they already know, with indications as to how and when they change from one to another. The following are two suggested lists, one for American bands and one for Middle Eastern:

A. *American Band:*

1. Enter to *Fiddler on the Roof* (Also, *Iskedara, Caravan*), Bright. On cue—

2. Segue to *Misirlou* (or *Taboo,* or both) Slow rhumba. On cue—

3. Drum solo, starting with slow rhumba and building to fast tempo. On cue—

4. Ensemble into *Fiddler*. On long turn—

5. End *Fiddler* with chord and drum roll.

B. *Middle Eastern Band:*

1. Enter to Sauda Sauda (Or Gezlarin, Hedy Lou) Fast. On cue—

2. Slow rhumba (Sulla Sunna, Bir Demet ya Semen) Slow On cue—

3. Cifte Telli, (improvised) Very slow. When rising from floor—

4. Drum solo into fast tempo. Follow dancer's movements. On cue—

5. Istemem Babajim (Or Daddy Lolo, Halvaji) Fast. On cue—

6. Rompi (Or Marinella) Fast Kashlimar (9/8) On Finale Drop—

7. End with chord.

APPENDIX II

COSTUMES

Being able to dance, and not having a costume to perform in is like the reverse of the old adage: "All dressed up and no place to go." In this case, you have some place to go, and nothing to wear! The following outline will tell you what a costume is, how it's made, and help you decide whether or not you really need it:

A. Costume Styles

A dancer's costume is one of the tools of her profession. It must be beautiful, and yet functional and practical since its entire purpose is to enhance the steps as well as to make the dancer look better. At this point, you would do well to forget the Hollywood costumes you have seen in the movies. They are created for "general purpose" dancers who learn choreographed routines for a given scene. The *real* belly dancer has her costumes made specifically for her (or makes her own) and dances in them in a variety of situations of lighting, backgrounds, and floor surfaces. In contrast to the Hollywood version, the real costume is very heavy. The hip-band weighs about seven pounds, while the lavishly beaded bra may weigh as much. The beads, in addition to being decorative, swing, and shimmy, and glisten with the movements of the dancer, so they make delicate steps (such as vibrations) visible from a distance. Elaborate and bulky headpieces are *out* for the real dancer. They look good, but are impossible to dance in. Ankle bells are effective in a short movie scene, but once the effect is achieved there is no way to turn them off, and they become a noisy irritation.

B. Making the Costume

1. *The skirt:* A basic skirt can be made of seven yards of a filmy material (usually nylon chiffon) though ten yards will make a more lavish one. The skirt is a beautiful addition to your practice session, since you can wear it over your leotard or body shirt. For this reason, it is wise to select a color which will complement your practice outfit. To make the skirt refer to the illustration and follow the steps below:

a. Measure hips, and length from hip-line to one inch below ankle.

b. Follow the diagram in cutting the skirt. After cutting you should have four pieces of fabric. One will be used for the front panel and three for the back.

c. Sew the three half-circles together to make the back panel.

d. Attach the back panel to *one side* of the hip-line of the front panel.

e. Hold the skirt around your hips, where it will be, and gather the material to fit snugly.

f. From excess material (from cutting) cut a one inch wide band, allowing for seams, and attach to hip-line of skirt.

g. Attach heavy-duty hook and eye for closing.

h. Hem bottom edge of skirt, and trim if desired.

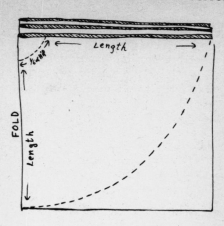

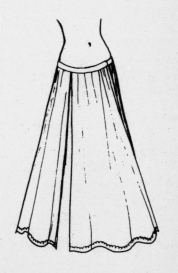

2. *The bra:*

a. Buy a bra with hard-shell cups (evening type).

b. Buy enough fabric (glistening satin, or silver or gold lamé) to cover bra and hip-band; about 3/4 yard. Also buy trim for bra and hip-band: jewels, beads, costume coins, etc. You can also use odds and ends of old jewelry you have around the house. Sequins can be used instead of beads, are easier to sew on, and can be purchased at the five-and-ten.

c. Remove the shoulder and back straps from bra.

d. Cover bra cups smoothly with the fabric.

e. Make new straps from cover fabric. Attach to cups using heavy-duty hooks and eyes for closing.

f. Straps are usually attached "halter style."

g. Refer to bra illustrations, create your own design, and trim bra and straps.

h. Line bra if you wish, and attach padding if necessary.

3. *The hip-band:*

a. Study the styles in the illustrations.

b. Buy approximately 1/2 yard of stiff pellon fabric.

c. From a large piece of paper (brown wrapping paper) cut a strip about 8 inches wide, and long enough to go around your hips. Trim to the desired shape, allowing overlap on the side where it will close.

d. Doubling the pellon, if you wish to add bulk and strength, transfer the pattern to the fabric. Also transfer pattern to material remaining from covering bra, leaving at least one inch all around for seam allowance.

e. Place the cover fabric over the pellon, and baste underneath.

f. Add trim, heavy-duty hooks and eyes, and line if you wish.

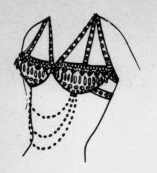
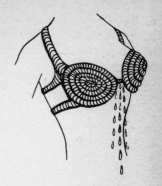
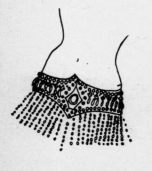
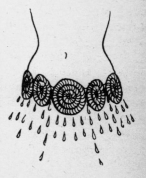

4. *The veil:*

a. The veil consists of approximately 2-1/4 yards of filmy fabric, which may be the same as the skirt if you wish.

b. Hem edges and trim if desired.

c. Study diagrams for ways of draping veil.

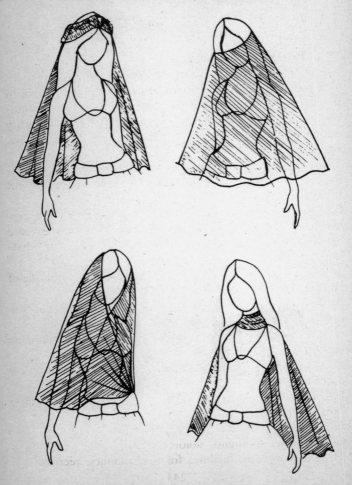

APPENDIX III

PUTTING ON A SHOW

The following outline is intended to be used as a guide in preparing for a major social function, such as a fund-raising dinner or organization banquet. But, it is easily adaptable for use in planning a small party in your home. In either case, plan ahead!

1. *Date and time:* Select a day when there are no conflicting events, especially religious observances (check out faiths other than your own!).

2. *Choosing the place:* In addition to meeting halls, restaurants, and catering houses, there are always the more exciting possibilities of boat rides and picnics. But whatever you choose, keep the following in mind:

A. Size; enough room for all, but not so large (and costly) that you can't fill it.

B. Food facilities; adequate and clean; check out the kitchen yourself.

C. Viewing; not too many pillars and posts; platform or bandstand a must.

D. Cost; shop around and compare prices; get *complete* cost list.

E. Location; easy to get to for all; public transportation runs at all hours.

F. Licensing; licensed for entertainment, liquor.

G. Lighting; spotlights, colored lights.

H. Sound system; facilities for microphones, records.

I.   Security; guards or police provided.

J.   Checking; adequate, safe checking for coats.

3.   *Assistants:* Be sure you have enough help. Don't underestimate problems!

A. Performers; make sure amateurs are prepared; contract professionals.

B. Music and musicians; records; if live, contract early; call union for scales.

C.   Cooks.

D.   Waiters

E.   Doormen, ticket takers, coat checkers.

4.   *Food:* Supply it yourself, cater it, or pot-luck. Typical Middle Eastern foods:

A. Dolma; stuffed grape leaves; comes ready made in cans.

B. Feta; white sheet or goat's-milk cheese.

C. Pastitso; baked macaroni Greek style; easy and cheap.

D. Baklava; thin pastry leaves with syrup and crushed walnuts; very rich.

E. Pita; flat Syrian bread.

F. Shishkebab; lamb marinated in coriander, mint, wine, etc.; cooked over coals.

G. Pilaf; rice or wheat cooked in broth.

H. Tabouli; salad of wheat, lemon juice, parsley, tomato.

I. Liquor; Ouzo; Greek brandy; retsina and red wine.

J. Coffee; Turkish and American.

K. Spinach pies.

L. Greek olives, pickles, etc.

M. Greek meat balls; kifte.

N. Roast lamb

O. Chicken, many Middle Eastern styles.

P. Fruit; dates; figs; pistachio nuts.

5.   *Decorations:* Travel posters; low tables with cushions; wrap posts with paper to create palm-tree effect; paint designs on windows with water paint; favors for guests such as fezes for men, veils for ladies, small tambourines.

Decorations can be rented. When using paper or flammable cloth, be sure to obey all fire laws!

6. *Tickets:* Plan whether to have tickets or pay at door. Reservations, if any.

7. *Activities:* Keep things moving; keep cliques from forming; include something everyone can participate in, such as folk-dancing; keep to a schedule, don't let speeches run too long; don't allow people to become stuffed with food and saturated with drink before putting on entertainment!

APPENDIX IV

EXERCISE CHART

BEGINNER

	Body Types 1 2 3 4 5 6	Other Benefits
Step 17		
ARM CIRCLE	X X	Shoulders, upper-arms
Variation (1)		Tension and release
Variation (1)		Control
Step 18		
PARALLEL ARM CIRCLE	X X X	Arms, shoulders, chest, upper back
Variation (1)		Control
Step 19		
KNEELING PARALLEL ARM CIRCLE	X X X	Shoulders, thighs, mid-section
Variation (2)		Entire torso!
Step 20		
FIGURE 8 OF HANDS	X X X X X X	Especially good for older women in toning skin of hands
Variation (1)		Upper-arms, shoulders
Step 21		
ALTERNATING FIGURE 8 OF HANDS WITH THORAX TWIST	X X X X X X	Waist through upper torso
Step 22		
TURKISH ARM POSE	X X	Isometric; shoulders and upper-arms
Step 23		
HIP EXTENSION	X	Hips, thighs
Step 24		
HEAD SLIDE AND HEAD CIRCLE	X X X X X X	Head, neck; excellent for double chin
Step 25		
HIP CIRCLE	X X	Hips, waist
Step 26		
FORWARD DIP AND CONTRACTION	X X X	Great for waist!

247

	Body Types						Other Benefits
	1	2	3	4	5	6	
Step 27 STEP—POINT—STEP	X		X	X			Coordination!
Variation (2)							Legs!
Step 28 VEIL ARM CIRCLE	X	X	X	X	X		Grace! coordination!
Variation (1)							Entire torso!
Step 29 BASIC WALK	X		X	X			Legs, thighs, stamina, grace
Variation (1)							Coordination, rhythm
Step 29A BASIC GLIDING WALK	X		X	X			Balance, poise
Variation (2)							Thighs!
Step 30 KNEE SLIDE	X		X	X			Thighs!!!!
Step 31 FINGER RIPPLE	X	X	X	X	X		Older women!
INTERMEDIATE STEPS							
Step 32 PIVOT BOUNCE			X	X		X	Thighs, lower back, mid-section
Step 33 SNAKE ARMS			X		X	X	Shoulders, upper-arms
Step 34 CLASSIC ARMS			X		X	X	Shoulders, upper-arms
Step 35 HINDOO ARM STEP	X	X	X	X	X		Arms, back, thighs
Step 36 UNDULATING ARCH AND CONTRACTION	X	X	X	X	X		Mid-section, particularly women after pregnancy
Variation (1)							Abdomen!!!
Step 37 HIP ROLL	X	X	X	X	X		Hips, mid-section
Step 38 HIP THRUST	X		X	X			Hips, mid-section
Step 38A HIP THRUST PIVOT TURN	X		X	X			Hips, thighs
Step 39 HIP THRUST WITH DEEP KNEE-BEND	X		X	X			Waist, hips, thighs, calves
Step 40 ANATOLIAN HIP MOVEMENT	X		X	X			Calves, thighs, waist
Variation (1)							Calves, thighs, waist!!!
Step 41 FLOOR DESCENT	X	X	X	X	X	X	Thighs, calves, balance and control!!!
Step 42 FLOOR DESCENT WITH UNDULATING ARCH AND CONTRACTION	X	X	X	X	X	X	Strenuous! entire body!

	Body Types						Other Benefits
	1	2	3	4	5	6	
Step 43							
BASIC KASHLIMAR	X	X	X	X	X	X	Entire body!!! coordination!
Variation (1)							Legs!
Step 44							
4/4 WALTZ	X	X	X	X	X	X	Mid-section; increases flexibility of abdomen!
Step 45							
FLOOR BACK-BEND	X	X	X	X	X	X	Very strenuous!!! thighs, back, abdomen
Step 46							
STEP—POINT—TURN	X	X	X	X	X	X	Mild! entire body
Variation (1)							Balance!
ADVANCED STEPS							
Step 47							
SHOULDER SHIMMY			X			X	Shoulders!
Step 48							
OASIS FLOOR LIFT	X			X	X		Hips, thighs, shoulders
Variation (2)							Arms, shoulders!
Step 49							
BELLY ROLL				X			Abdomen!!
Step 50							
DOUBLE HIP THRUST	X			X	X		Hips, legs, abdomen
Variation (3)							Legs! entire body
Step 51							
HOP WITH DOUBLE FLEX	X	X	X	X	X	X	Mid-section, flexibility
Step 52							
ABDOMINAL BODY SWIVEL				X			Hips, abdomen
Step 53							
HIP TWIST HEEL AND TOE				X			Hips, abdomen
Step 54							
PELVIC FLUTTER	X			X	X		Thighs, abdomen
Step 55							
KNEELING HIP EXTENSION	X			X			Thighs, hips, waist
Step 56							
HIP SHIMMY	X	X	X	X	X	X	Strenuous! arms, shoulders, stamina
Step 57							
VIBRATIONS	X	X	X	X	X	X	Control, relaxation.
Step 58							
HIP SKIP	X	X	X	X	X	X	Entire body, stamina
Variation (2)							Legs! coordination
Step 59							
STEP SLIDE	X	X	X	X	X	X	Legs
Step 59A							
PIVOT TURN	X	X	X	X	X	X	Entire body! balance!
Step 60							
9/8 ROCK	X	X	X	X	X	X	Legs, stamina
Variation (2)							Waist

	1	2	3	4	5	6	Other Benefits
Body Types							
Step 61 **TURKISH TRAVEL**	X	X	X	X	X		Legs, coordination, timing
Variation (1)							Calves!
Step 62 **KNEELING TORSO SPIN**	X	X	X	X	X	X	Strenuous! stamina!
Step 63 **ARCHED STANDING BACK-BEND**		X		X	X		Strenuous! thighs, back, abdomen
Step 64 **CONTRACTED STANDING BACK-BEND**		X		X	X		Strenuous!!! thighs! back! abdomen! balance!!!
Step 65 **DERVISH SPIN**	X	X	X	X	X	X	Balance!
Step 66 **FORWARD FIGURE 8 OF TORSO**	X	X	X	X	X	X	Mid-section!
Step 67 **9/8 CHA CHA**		X		X	X		Coordination
Step 68 **DEBKE STEP**	X	X	X	X	X	X	Coordination
Variation (2)							Abdomen
Step 69 **HIP ROLL DIP**		X		X	X		Back! thighs! legs! balance!
Step 70 **UNDULATING ARCH AND CONTRACTION WALK (CAMEL WALK)**	X	X	X	X	X	X	Entire torso, coordination, balance!
Variation (2)							Balance!
Step 71 **HIP CIRCLE WITH WALK**	X	X	X	X	X	X	Waist, balance, grace
Step 72 **HIP ROLL WITH WALK**	X	X	X	X	X	X	Waist, balance, poise
Step 73 **HUBBLE BUBBLE**		X		X	X		Strenuous! legs, thighs, hips, waist
Step 74 **DOUBLE HUBBLE BUBBLE**		X		X	X		Strenuous! legs, thighs, hips, waist
Step 75 **RUNNING STEP SHIMMY**		X		X	X		Strenuous! legs, stamina!
Step 76 **ARCH AND CONTRACTION PIVOT TURN**	X	X	X	X	X	X	Back!
Variation (2)							Abdomen!
Variation (3)							Back!!!
Step 77 **HIP CIRCLE WITH TURN**	X	X	X	X	X	X	Waist, hips, balance

	Body Types						Other Benefits
	1	2	3	4	5	6	
Step 78 BELLY FLUTTER				X			Abdomen!
Step 79 REVERSE ARCH AND CONTRACTION				X			Abdomen, back
Step 80 STEP—POINT—ARCH— EXTEND	X	X	X	X	X	X	Strenuous!!! back! legs! abdomen! hips!
Step 81 ARABIC COFFEE MILL	X	X	X	X	X	X	Abdomen!
Step 82 HIP TWIST OPEN KNEE-BEND Variation (1)	X	X	X	X	X	X	Strenuous! legs! hips! waist! Strenuous!!! legs!!
Step 83 BERBER KNEE WALK	X	X	X	X	X	X	Legs! thighs! calves!
Step 84 GYPSY HOP TURN	X	X	X	X	X	X	Strenuous! stamina! balance
Step 85 FINALE DROP		X		X	X		Legs, coordination, balance

INDEX OF STEPS

Abdominal Body Swivel (Step 52), 169
Alternating Figure 8 of Hands with Thorax Twist (Step 21), 92
Anatolian Hip Movement (Step 40), 133
Arabic Coffee Mill (Step 81), 214
Arch and Contraction Pivot Turn (Step 76), 207
Arched Standing Back-Bend (Step 63), 187
Arm Circle (Step 17), 84

Basic Kashlimar (Step 43), 138
Basic Walk (Step 29), 106
Belly Flutter (Step 78), 210
Belly Roll (Step 49), 163
Berber Knee Walk (Step 83), 218

Classic Arms (Step 34), 118
Contracted Standing Back-Bend (Step 64), 188

Debke Step (Step 68), 194
Dervish Spin (Step 65), 190
Double Hip Thrust (Step 50), 165
Double Hubble Bubble (Step 74), 204

Figure 8 of Hands (Step 20), 90
Finale Drop (Step 85), 221
Finger Ripple (Step 31), 109

Floor Back-Bend (Step 45), 145

Floor Descent (Step 41), 135

Floor Descent with Undulating Arch and Contraction (Step 42), 137

Forward Dip and Contraction (Step 26), 100

Forward Figure 8 of Torso (Step 66), 191

4/4 Waltz (Step 44), 142

Gypsy Hop-Turn (Step 84), 220

Head Slide and Head Circle (Step 24), 96

Heel Bounce (Step 16), 82

Hindoo Arm Step (Step 35), 120

Hip Circle (Step 25), 98

Hip Circle with Turn (Step 77), 209

Hip Circle with Walk (Step 71), 201

Hip Extension (Step 23), 95

Hip Roll (Step 37), 126

Hip Roll Dip (Step 69), 196

Hip Roll with Walk (Step 72), 202

Hip Shimmy (Step 56), 175

Hip Skip (Step 58), 178

Hip Slide (Step 9), 75

Hip Swivel (Step 10), 76

Hip Thrust (Step 38), 129

Hip Thrust with Deep Knee-Bend (Step 39), 132

Hip Twist—Heel and Toe (Step 53), 171

Hip Twist Open Knee-Bend (Step 82), 216

Hop with Double Flex (Step 51), 168

Hubble Bubble (Step 73), 203

Knee Dip and Twist (Step 12), 78

Knee Slide (Step 30), 108

Knee-Bend Holding Contraction (Step 15), 81

Knee-Bend with Arched Back (Step 14), 80

Kneeling Hip Extension (Step 55), 173

Kneeling Parallel Arm Circle (Step 19), 88
Kneeling Sit-up (Step 13), 79
Kneeling Torso Spin (Step 62), 186

Large Circle of Shoulders (Step 3), 69

9/8 Cha Cha (Step 67), 192
9/8 Rock (Step 60), 182

Oasis Floor Lift (Step 48), 161

Parallel Arm Circle (Step 18), 86
Pelvic Flutter (Step 54), 173
Pelvic Tilt (Step 11), 77
Pivot Bounce (Step 32), 113
Pivot Turn (Step 59A), 181

Reverse Arch and Contraction (Step 79), 210
Rib-Cage Circle (Step 7), 73
Rib-Cage Extension (Step 6), 72
Running Step Shimmy (Step 75), 205

Shoulder Shimmy (Step 47), 160
Shoulder Slant (Step 2), 68
Shoulder Slide (Step 1), 66
Shoulder Thrust (Step 5), 71
Small Shoulder Circles (Step 4), 70
Snake Arms (Step 33), 115
Spinal Flex (Step 8), 74
Step—Point—Arch—Extend (Step 80), 213
Step—Point—Step (Step 27), 101
Step—Point—Turn (Step 46), 148
Step—Slide (Step 59), 181

Turkish Arm Pose (Step 22), 94
Turkish Travel (Step 61), 184

Undulating Arch and Contraction (Step 36), 123
Undulating Arch and Contraction Walk (Camel Walk) (Step 70), 198

Veil Arm Circle (Standing and Kneeling) (Step 28), 210
Vibrations (Step 57), 177